The Wet Engine

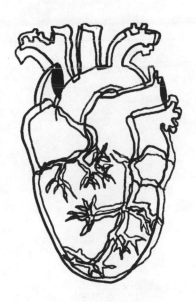

The Wet Engine
exploring the mad wild miracle of the heart

by Brian Doyle

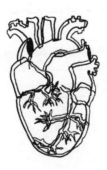

Oregon State University Press • Corvallis

The paper in this book meets the guidelines for permanence
and durability of the Committee on Production Guidelines
for Book Longevity of the Council on Library Resources
and the minimum requirements of the American National
Standard for Permanence of Paper for Printed Library
Materials Z39.48-1984.

Library of Congress Cataloging-in-Publication Data
Doyle, Brian, 1956 Nov. 6-
The wet engine : exploring the mad wild miracle of the heart
/ by Brian Doyle.
   p. cm.
   ISBN 978-0-87071-653-9
   e-ISBN 978-0-87071-654-6
1. Heart—Religious aspects—Christianity. 2. Heart—
Diseases—Religious aspects—Christianity. I. Title.
BT741.3.D69 2005
241'.4—dc22   2005000194

First published in 2005 by Paraclete Press.
First Oregon State University Press edition 2012
Printed in the United States of America

Oregon State University Press
121 The Valley Library
Corvallis OR 97331-4501
541-737-3166 • fax 541-737-3170
http://osupress.oregonstate.edu

For David McIrvin & Linda Dickson McIrvin

Contents

Foreword

The convergence of the professional and personal is never neat or easy. As a nurse now in my fourth decade of professional life, I've learned to navigate the rough channel between personal and professional, neatly compartmentalizing my knowledge and responsibilities. The joy of my discipline is that my professional purpose—caring—is deeply connected to my personal values. Beyond that, though, there is endless separation and compartmentalization. Roles, responsibilities, and even language signal my nursing engagement; under it all, of course, is that core of caring.

But Brian Doyle does not help at *all* in this matter. His book about the human heart doesn't fit nicely in my library, or in how I've related to hearts in the past. Brian won't stick to one script or the other. Nor will he allow us to forget that these boundaries that we erect among who we are in our roles as patient, professional, or parent really don't work. And, in real matters of the heart, they collide in wonderful and painful ways.

The Wet Engine is about *all* matters of the heart, and it is about one particular boy's heart—Liam, Brian's son. The physical and metaphysical are connected here, as are insights about what breaks and heals hearts. For one whose cardiac disease and healing has lived in the realm of health and medicine, these insights require reflection and rethinking. Fortunately, though, *The Wet Engine* is both manual and map, allowing us to learn the heart's mechanics, while guiding us on an exploration of the beauty and mystery of what lies within each of us. Brian clearly knows—and helps us learn—that all matters of the heart are, indeed, matters of God.

At its core, this book is about relationships—with family, God, and our own hearts. It is also about thinking differently about everything we've thought of or believed about the subject.For me, the nurse, this book is about wholeness and hearing the beat of the human heart as a whisper of divinity. What a wonderful gift from the deep and generous heart of father and author Brian Doyle.

Marla Salmon
Dean of Nursing
University of Washington
Seattle, Washington

Introduction

My son Liam was born nine years ago. He looked like a cucumber on steroids. He was fat and bald and round. He looked healthy as a horse. He wasn't. He was missing a chamber in his heart, which was a problem, as you need four chambers for smooth conduct through this vale of fears and tears, and he only had three chambers, so pretty soon he had an open-heart surgery, during which doctors cut him open and iced down his heart and shut it down for an hour or so while they worked on repair.

That was when he was about six months old. I don't remember much about that time. It all rushed past like a pain train.

Then when he was about eighteen months old he had another open-heart surgery, during which they did all that again, and what I most remember from that time is his grinning face receding down the hallway as he was carried toward the bone shears by a sweet quiet doctor. I'll always remember that. His face was so round. His face bounced up and down a little on the doctor's thin shoulder. He smiled at me at the very end of the corridor, just before he and the doctor turned the corner, and I thought maybe that was going to be the last time I ever saw that big fat face smiling at me, and that was when I saw pain and death leering at me closer than I ever saw them before. That was a cold moment. I'll always remember that.

*

Well, that wasn't the last time I saw my boy Liam, I am almighty happy to report, and now he's pretty much fine, although he's stubborn as a stone, and a grouch in the morning, and he gets tired more than he admits, and eventually he will have to get a new heart altogether, and he has been told by his genius heart doctor that he shouldn't play football or run marathons, neither of which I think he was thinking of doing anyway, the kid being a basketball nut first and foremost.

Now he is nine years old. He's one of the most interesting and gentle people I ever met, and I am awfully glad that he didn't die.

His surgeries were years ago now, and his next surgery, the big one, when they take out his creaky old heart and pop in a new one, is ten or twenty or thirty years in the future. Don't worry about it, says his genius heart doctor, by then we'll have figured out something waaaay better than transplants.

So I don't worry about it, much. Sometimes I do worry about it a lot but I don't tell my wife because I know she worries too and I have learned there are some things, a lot of things, with which you shouldn't worry a wife.

But the days pass in their swirl and whirl and swing and song, and every day he doesn't die again, and that knocks me out.

*

So everything seems fairly normal these days. Liam runs around like an insane dorky gawky goofy heron and rides his bike and shoots hoop and skateboards and swings and punches out his brother and snarls at his sister and refuses to make his bed but he does actually set the table every night and help cook dinner sometimes and he does his homework pretty carefully when he doesn't leave his backpack at school and he eats more yogurt and grapes and blueberries than anyone I ever saw and his hair won't stay combed no matter what and he's a really good artist and he makes perfect pancakes and he is almost all the time a cheerful entertaining kind-hearted mammal whose company I really enjoy.

He gets sick and he gets well and his knees are knobby and he just got a perfect score on his spelling test yesterday and the days and nights pass in their magic music, each more beautiful than the last, each one so filled with joy and pain and shouting and sadness and mud and angst and dishes and milk and jam and bills and newspapers and underwear and coffee filters and insurance payments and flat tires and rain and crows that I want to weep with helpless happiness sometimes for no reason that I can understand one bit at all.

*

But not a day goes by, not one, that I do not think of my son tiny and round and naked and torn open and heart-chilled and swimming somewhere between death and life; and every day I think of the young grinning intense mysterious heart doctor who saved his life; and for years now I have wanted to try to write that most unwriteable man down, to tell a handful of the thousands of stories that whirl around him like brilliant birds, to report a tiny percentage of the people he has saved and salved, and so thank him in some way I don't fully understand, and also thank the Music that made him and me and my son and all of us; and somehow it seems to me that the writing down of a handful of those stories will *matter* in the world, be a sort of crucial chant or connective tissue between writer and readers, all of us huddled singing under the falling bombs and stars; and more and more over the years I have become absorbed and amazed at the heart itself, the wet engine of us all, and how it works and doesn't work, and what it means, and how we use it so easily and casually as a metaphor for the extraordinary loves and agonies that course through us like muscular raging rivers; so finally I sit my raggedy self down and write this lean book, as a sort of prayer of thanks that my son is alive and stubborn as a stone, that there are such complicated and graceful people as Doctor Dave, that there are such mysterious and incalculably holy things as hammering hearts, and that they power such mysterious and holy and wild things as us.

*

Look, I don't know much, but I know these things uncontrovertibly and inarguably:

One: stories matter waaaaay more than we know.

Two: all stories are, in some form, prayers.

Three: love is the story and the prayer that matters the most.

So: here are some stories and prayers, and they are all about love, and I hope they matter to you too.

Brian Doyle

1. The Infinite Number of Things
That Can Go Wrong with the Hearts of New People

Doctor Dave McIrvin is slight and thin and intense and smiling and one of those puzzling human creatures who while they are talking to you seem to have all the time in the universe, and look you right in the eye, and answer your questions directly and straightforwardly, and listen to what you say, and don't listen impatiently waiting for you to finish what foolish thing *you* are saying so they can tell you what wise thing *they* know, but as soon as you are finished talking to Dave he is gone like a cat. He just is *gone*. It's the most amazing thing you ever saw. Because he is a doctor he almost always is wearing green scrubs so if you pay attention and watch carefully when he begins to be gone you see a greenish whir and blur in the air, topped by Dave's grin, and then the vision and Dave are both gone, and you are standing there thinking that old Lewis Carroll knew what he was talking about when he invented the Cheshire Cat.

*

Dave is a pediatric cardiologist. Kids call him Doctor Dave, or Doccor Dave, or just Dave. One time a kid called him a cardio pediologist. He looks like he might be thirty years old but he came into the world in California fifty years ago. His dad ran a pest-control service and his mom helped his dad run the pest-control service and she also raised Dave and his older brother Art.

Was Dave a good boy? I ask his mom.

He was *not* a good boy, she says, firmly. He would do exactly the thing you told him *not* to do. That's just how he was.

She says this very politely but precisely. She loves her younger son with a love patient and powerful but she does not forget, for example, what she refers to darkly as *the motorcycle incident*, of which the less said here the better.

Everybody gets fascinated by something when they are young and some people pursue their fascination with tenacity all their lives and Dave pursued his, which was biology. He was fascinated by how living things worked and didn't work. In college, in California, he studied how living things worked and didn't work and then in graduate school, in Oregon, he studied how living things worked and didn't work, and then he decided he wanted to be a doctor, to fix living things that weren't working very well.

He applied to the best medical schools in America but none of them agreed that he should enroll in their august halls of learning. He was counseled to wait a year and try again, to spend another year in graduate school and earn even more impressive grades and do a creative science or service project that would add value to his application, but Dave is a brisk and stubborn man, and he wanted to be in medical school right then, so he applied to, and was accepted by, Saint George's University School of Medicine, on the island of Grenada, in the West Indies.

*

Grenada, the Spice Island, is famous for clove and cinnamon. It is famous for nutmeg and ginger. It is famous for its eccentric former prime minister, the Right Honorable Sir Eric Gairy, who led his tiny nation to independence from England in

1974, who communicated regularly with extraterrestrials, who once told *Time* magazine that his opponents were negativity and he was positivity, and who told reporters that when his opponents hated him he replied by sending out waves of love to them. And Grenada is famous for being the smallest nation ever invaded by the United States of America. It was attacked by the United States Army at dawn on October 25, 1983, when more than a thousand Army Rangers parachuted onto the island by order of President Ronald Reagan, who wished to dismantle the Marxist government that had itself taken power by bloody coup the week before.

The Army Rangers landed at Point Salines, on the island's south side, and soon swept over the island toward Saint George's University's three campuses, where they secured the safety of 599 American medical students who were, says Dave, not in danger at all, and paying the same amount of attention to the invasion that they had paid to the revolution four years before, which is to say none. The revolution four years before had caused the medical students to miss morning classes, which they made up that night.

By the time of the invasion Dave had graduated and moved along in his ambition to be a professional fixer of living things, but he remembers the revolution well. It lasted about half an hour, says Dave, after which a young Grenadian lawyer, Maurice Bishop, with whom Dave had played billiards at the Sugar Mill, the local bar, seized power from the Right Honorable Sir Eric Gairy, who moved along to New York City. The medical students were not especially sad to see Sir Eric leave, as he was fond of trying to pick up female medical students at the Sugar Mill.

During the revolution, says Dave, the medical students played softball and went swimming. Dave liked to swim in the lucid waters off Grenada, even after meeting a huge barracuda the first time he dove in, and he liked playing softball, especially with the cheerful Cuban laborers who were building an airport near campus, but he liked most of all to go for runs, to burn off the tension of medical school, to fly through the warm salt air of the island, to stop thinking, to just float. Often when he ran he would be followed by a dozen or so Grenadian schoolchildren in their school uniforms, giggling at the thin white man running with the big grin. Dave would stop and wait for them and when they caught up to him he would take the hand of one child, who would take the hand of another child, and so on down the line of children the handholding would go like an electric current, and they would all run down the road hand in hand, Dave grinning and the children giggling and the bookbags and pigtails of the children flapping and flopping and flying through the moist spicy air.

*

Dave finished first in his class at Saint George's University's School of Medicine and graduated on Halloween of 1982 and then began his pediatric residency at Baylor College of Medicine and Texas Children's Hospital, both in Houston, Texas.

One night early in 1984 the nurse on duty in the intensive care unit at Texas Children's Hospital had an infant patient named Joshua in respiratory distress. She paged the resident on call. The resident on call had the flu and was asleep in the on-call room but within seconds of her page he showed up, brisk and alert, although he had pillow lines on his face and his hair was a mess. He fixed Joshua's breathing and chaffed the duty nurse and went back to sleep and that's how Linda Dickson met Dave McIrvin and vice versa.

I liked him right off, she says. There was something different about him.

She caught my attention from the first minute we spoke, he says. There was just something different about her.

Two months later he asked her to dinner, and a year later he asked her if she would maybe like to get a house together, which invitation she found a little presumptuous and was about to refuse, when he added that they could also get a dog together, which invitation she found alluring and did not refuse, so one dog later they were married in a tiny church on the coast of Maine, and they have been married now for five dogs.

*

Linda and her brother grew up in Texas. Her mother was a terrific piano player and her father was an engineer. Her brother became a banker and Linda went to college. She studied psychology at the University of Texas and became a social worker but she grew weary of being a social worker. She went to law school for a semester and hated it and went to nursing school and loved it and she became a nurse. She was a staff nurse and a teaching nurse and a nurse manager, all in the pediatric intensive care unit, and then an emergency nurse and an outpatient nurse. After seventeen years of nursing she found herself working full-time part-time shifts, sometimes twenty hours at a stretch, for no benefits, and very often her long shifts and Dave's long shifts meant that they hardly saw each other for days on end, and so she retired and began to write a murder mystery.

Ever since I was a little girl I wanted to be a writer and now I am a writer, she says. It's not for me to say if I am any *good* as a writer, but I like to write and I understand my characters better and better the more I write about them, which seems like a good sign to me. I don't know how other people write books but I find that I have to get all the way to the end of the story before I can see it clearly enough to rewrite it, so I have written the book several times, I suppose. But every time I write it it's a different book. So I have either written one book five times or five books once each.

*

One time when Dave and I had just started dating, says Linda, I was working a night shift and we heard that Doctor Denton Cooley was going to do a heart transplant that night. My unit was very slow that night so I asked my charge nurse if I could go watch the transplant. She told me to stay for the whole thing. Dave was on call and asked me to page him when I heard the heart had arrived. He wanted to watch too. A respiratory therapist told me when the heart arrived. Respiratory therapists travel all over hospitals and carry all the news to everyone. So in the wee hours of the morning Dave and I sat in the dark for hours over the dome that looks directly down into the patient's chest, and we watched the surgeons take the old heart out and put the new one in, and that was a miracle. That was a magical night. I'll always remember it. When the new heart started beating, it was ... magic.

*

Another time when we were in Texas, says Linda, when Dave was doing his pediatrics residency, all the residents did something called continuity clinic, which is basically following the same kids through all three years of your residency. The kids were chronic patients, with tracheotomies, feeding tubes, etc. These kids basically alternated living at home and being in the hospital. So one year Dave and some of the other residents decided to take the kids to the circus. This was a pretty big deal, involving special permission and waivers, transportation for wheelchairs, oxygen, etc. One girl had the condition called Ondine's Curse, her breathing was impaired and they had to ambu bag her the whole time; an ambu bag is attached to oxygen and you squeeze it with your hand to breathe for a patient when she's temporarily off her ventilator.

But they pulled the circus trip off. Dave likes to talk about it. One kid had a fistula, so when he ate ice cream it came out the side of his throat, but he was in absolute ecstasy. I always loved that story.

*

After Dave's three years as a pediatric resident, and instructor, and Linda's concurrent years as a nurse, Dave looked for work as a pediatric cardiologist, and was offered a position at Maine Medical Center, in Portland, Maine. The Great State of Maine appealed to Linda as well, so she and Dave and their dogs moved to Maine, and Dave embarked on his career in analysis and repair of the infinite number of things that can go wrong with the hearts of new people.

One day I ask him why he chose this particular field of medicine, in which the emotional ocean is incomprehensibly deep and roiling.

I figured, where do you have saves?, he says. Where do you have cures? Where can you work with children with your hands? Where do you have an immediate impact? Where could I do things that were unimaginable fifty years ago? Where could I help fix problems that were devastating and fatal fifty years ago? I wanted to work with kids but I didn't want to be a sore-throat doctor and I didn't want to be a surgeon and I didn't want to be a laboratory doctor. So I went into hearts.

Good answer, Dave, I say.

I've thought about it some, he says.

*

Two years after Dave and Linda and the dogs moved to Maine the phone rang and a doctor named Doug King offered Dave a job. This was with a small independent concern called the Children's Cardiac Center of Oregon, which consisted mostly of Doug King and the doctor who had founded the company, Martin Lees, an Englishman who had been the first pediatric cardiologist in Oregon. Lees and King were so busy that they could hardly spit and they needed a third pediatric cardiologist bad. Dave and Linda talked it over and for all that they loved living on the coast of Maine there were pressing and alluring reasons to move: the job entailed far more pioneering and risky challenges, and Linda could easily find work as a nurse, and Oregon was a land of surpassing rugged and riveting wilderness outside Portland, and Oregon was much closer to California, where Dave's folks lived, than Maine was, and no further away from Texas, where Linda's folks lived, than Maine was.

So they moved to Oregon.

In the thirteen years since he and Linda moved to Oregon, Dave has seen some seven thousand patients, ages zero to fifty, most of them from Oregon and Washington and Alaska and British Columbia but some of them from Colombia, Panama, Mexico, Venezuela, Siberia, the Sudan, China, Russia, Iran, Latvia, Bulgaria, Armenia, and Truk, which is an island so far away from Dave's office that to fly from Truk to Oregon you have to fly through today into yesterday. He has diagnosed every sort of heart malfunction and malformation there is, and he has spent more than forty thousand hours of his life pondering the repair of the hearts of his patients, but of those many hours and patients the hours he spent on one particular pediatric patient matter the most to me, for that patient was and is my miraculous complex odd unique son, who was born missing a chamber in his heart.

I don't know about you, but when I am really frightened by something, really filled with fear, really terrified, I find myself getting utterly absorbed by the tiniest details. I think it's a form of emotional defense or something—if you can focus on the infinitesimal, then the vast can't get a good grip on you, can't get its hooks in, can't get its pincers into play.

Anyway, when Liam turned out to have most of a heart instead of all of a heart, and there was an emergency medical team ready at his birth because they thought he might die right off, and then Dave explained the horrifying nature of the operations that would have to be performed, well, I got utterly absorbed in the vast details of his tiny heart. I read everything I could find, I asked a million questions, I hid in the thicket of facts and diagrams, and maybe that was a coward's way of dealing with the world, I don't know, but all these years later I remember many of those facts and diagrams, and they fascinate me still.

So as some strange act of celebration or prayer or testimony, let us wander into the wet engine, and apprehend the miracle and study the mystery, and be agog and agape at what has been so wondrously wrought in the meat beneath the bone of your chest.

2. Heartchitecture

Let us contemplate, you and I, the bloody electric muscle. Let us consider it from every angle. Let us remove it from its bony cage, its gristly case, and hold it to the merciless light, and turn it glinting this way and that, and look at it as if we have never seen it before, because we never *have* seen it before, not like this. Let us think carefully about the throb of its relentless tissue. Let us ponder it as the wet engine from which comes all the music we know. Let us contemplate the thousand ways it fails and the few ways it does not fail. Let us gawk at the brooding genius of its architecture. Let us consider it as the most crucial and amazing house, with its four rooms and meticulous plumbing and protein walls and chambered music. Let us dream of blood and pulse and ebb and flow. Let us consider tide and beat and throb and hum. Let us unweave the web of artery and vein, the fluttering jetties of the valves, the coursing of ions from cell to cell, the sodium that is your soul, the potassium that is your personality, the calcium that is your character.

*

Consider the astounding journey your blood embarks upon as it enters the pumping station of your heart. In a healthy heart, a heart that works as it has been designed to work over many millions of years by its creative and curious and tireless and nameless holy wild silent engineer, blood that has been plucked and shucked of its oxygen by the body straggles back into the right atrium, the capacious gleaming lobby of the heart.

This tired blood, dusty veteran of an immense and exhausting journey, shuffles forward to and through a small circular door in the wall, a door with three symmetrical flaps: the tricuspid valve.

This circular door opens into another big room, the right ventricle; but at the very instant the right ventricle is filled to capacity with tired blood the entire ventricle *contracts!*, slamming in on itself, and our tired heroes are sent flying through the pulmonary valve and thence into the pulmonary artery, which immediately branches, carrying the blood to the right and left lungs, and there, in the joyous airy countries of the blood vessels of the lungs, your blood is given fresh clean joyous oxygen!, gobs and slathers of it!, o sweet and delicious air!, as much as those heroic blood cells can hoist aboard their tiny cellular ships, and now they resume their endless journey, heading into the marshlands and swamps of the lungs, the capillary beds, which open into the small streams and creeks called venules, which are tributaries of the pulmonary veins, of which there are four, the four magic pulmonary rivers carrying your necessary elixir back to the looming holy castle of the heart, which they will enter this time through the left atrium, whose job is to disperse and assign the blood to the rest of the body, to send it on its quest and voyage and journey to the vast and mysterious wilderness that is you, and to tell that tale, of the journeys of your blood cells through the universe of you, would take a billion books, each alike, each utterly different.

*

But so much can go wrong. So much does go wrong. So many ways to go wrong. Aneurysm, angina, arrythmia, blockages and obstructions, ischmemias and infections, vascular and valvular failure, pericarditis and pressure problems, strokes and syndromes, the ways that hearts falter and fail are endless. They clog and stutter. They sigh and stop. They skip a beat. They lose the beat. Or they beat so fast and so madly that they endure electrical frenzies. One electrical frenzy is called circus movement: the electrical impulse leaves the rhythmic world of contraction-and-rest and enters a state of essentially continuous beat. A heart in circus movement may beat five hundred times a minute for as long as ninety seconds before it stops altogether and the person wrapped around that heart dies.

*

Consider those ninety seconds. A minute and a half. The fastest and last minute and a half of that one life. A minute and a half tipped forward into relentless irretrievable headlong final free fall. The heart sprinting toward oblivion, unable to rest, revving unto chaos; achieving, for the last ninety seconds of its working life, a state of such intense beat that it comes as close to beatlessness as it ever could while beating: until it ceases to beat.

*

Or think of the heart as a music machine—not a farfetched idea, for the heart runs on electric impulse and does so in a steady 4/4 rhythm. A musician friend of mine maintains that the 4/4 rhythm, standard in popular music, feels right, feels normal, because it is the pace of our hearts, the interior music we hear all day and all night. We are soaked in the song of the heart every hour of every year every life long.

Fill my heart with song, sings Frank Sinatra, and is your heart filled with pain?, sings Elvis Presley, and my heart will go on, sings Celine Dion, and open your heart, sings Elton John, and open your heart, sings Lenny Kravitz, and he had a heart of glass, sings Blondie, and I've been a miner for a heart of gold, sings Neil Young, and don't be blind heart of mine, rasps Bob Dylan, and why does my heart feel so bad, moans Moby, and put a little love in your heart, sings Annie Lennox, and everybody's got a hungry heart, roars Bruce Springsteen, and my heart still beats, sings Beyonce Knowles, and Lord with glowing heart I'd praise Thee, sang Francis Scott Key, and stop draggin' my heart around, snarls Tom Petty, and I got them broken heart blues, mumbled Sonny Boy Williamson, and I canna live without the inarticulate speech of the heart, sings the genius Van Morrison, and this is the last chance for hearts of stone, sings Southside Johnny Lyon, and lock me in your heart, sings Mandy Moore, and unchain my heart, sings Joe Cocker, and what would rock and pop and blues and gospel and jazz and soul and rap music do without this most necessary musical organ? Would there even be such a thing as pop music if there were no hearts to break and fill and unchain and hijack?

*

It weighs eleven ounces. It feeds a vascular system that comprises sixty thousand miles of veins and arteries and capillaries. It beats a hundred thousand times a day. It shoves two thousand gallons of blood through the body every day. It begins when a fetus is three weeks old and a cluster of cells begins to pulse with the cadence of that particular person, a music and rhythm and pace that will endure a whole lifetime. No one knows why the cluster of cells begins to pulse at that time or with that beat. These cells undergo what is called spontaneous depolarization. Channels inside these cells begin to leak sodium and the wash of sodium sparks the trading of potassium and calcium back and forth which inspires an electrical current which augmented is the beat of your heart. These cells are infectious, as it were; if you put them alongside any other type of cell in the body, they make the other cells beat to their beat.

*

The heart is the first organ to form. It is smaller than a comma when it begins and ends up bigger than a fist. Every cell in it is capable of pulsing. No one knows how that could be. The pulse begins when a baby is about twenty days old. No one knows quite why it happens then. The pulse then continues, on average, for about two billion pulses. No one knows why there are that many. Or that few. Why not one billion each? Why not twenty billion? Mayflies to mastodons, beetles to bison, prophets to poets, infants to those who commit infanticide, all are issued the same number of pulses to do with what they will. Tell me, asks the great quiet American poet Mary Oliver, what is it you plan to do with your one wild and precious life?

*

Consider the engineering of the heart. It begins life as a primitive hollow tube of tissue which bends and loops and twists and turns and envelops and overlaps and intricately creates itself as a heart, the wings and tendrils of tissue advancing and retreating, holes and spaces appearing, walls and valves constructing themselves according to a mysterious and extraordinary command and design, all this infinitesimal heartchitecture bathed in the one fluid in the ancient universe that can sustain the new wet machine: rich fresh blood from the mother, which she sends through the placenta to her developing child in oxygenated bursts to the new brain, the new heart, the rest of the body.

Here are some magic numbers: all mothers at all times past and present to all children developing under their hearts send 62 percent of placental blood to the new brain, 29 percent to the new body, and 9 percent to the heart. Hitler and Ho, Gandhi and Gautama, Mohammed and Maimonides, Mao and Moses, the Madonna and her mother, the Madonna and her Child: when they were fingers of flesh floating in their mothers, new ideas clinging to uterine walls, they received blood from their mothers in exactly the same doses.

*

In America these days one woman dies every minute of every day from a failed heart. More women die of failed hearts than men. Failed hearts kill more women and men than the next seven causes of death combined. The highest rate of death by failed heart is in Utah. The lowest rate is in Mississippi. More than four hundred babies are born every day with flawed hearts. Eight of every thousand babies are born with flawed hearts. One percent of all babies born all over the world are born with flawed hearts. Twenty percent of all babies born with flawed hearts will die before their first birthday.

*

Our body fluids contain about one percent salt, nowadays, very likely the exact salinity of whatever ancient sea we managed to crawl out of, a sea we could leave because we had learned, first of all, to contain it; and that sea is contained and remembered most crucially now in the heart, where salt sloshes back and forth between cells, forming the first thrum of the heartbeat, the first hint of the absolute and necessary note from which comes the salty song of You.

*

"Seat of the affections," thinks James Joyce's genius creature Leopold Bloom, standing by a new grave in *Ulysses*. "Broken heart. A pump after all, pumping thousands of gallons of blood every day. One fine day it gets bunged up; and there you are. Lots of them lying around here ... old rusty pumps ..."

*

Consider the economics of the heart, the industries that encircle it like pericardium. Diseases of the heart in America alone cost nearly $400 billion annually. More than half of that cost is health care for the damaged; the rest is estimated lost productivity from the damaged. Diseases of the heart in the world as a whole, over the course of a year, cost more than a trillion dollars. A trillion dollars is hard to imagine. It's hard to even write a trillion in mathematical notation. Fifteen zeroes is a lot of zeroes, so many that you have to organize them in little groups of three, using commas like fences. As if the zeroes were wild and unruly and would run off were they not corralled.

*

Nor does a trillion dollars tell any stories at all. It's a useless worthless number that way. It doesn't have any of the swirl and whirl of the heart. It doesn't tell you about the young mother in a village whose heart just stops in her sleep one night and her young son wakes up first in the morning and smiles at his mama and he figures he'll be a good boy and he gets the fire going and then kisses her to wake her up and she will be surprised and delighted at the excellent little fire he made and when she doesn't wake he kisses her again and then for the first time in his whole life he feels a naked shiver of fear in his heart.

It doesn't tell you about the girl who is a genius who spends her entire brief existence on the planet pale and gasping instead of being a genius.

It doesn't tell you about the million men and women and children in rural valleys and mountain redoubts and desert enclaves and ragged jungle clearings whose hearts could be regulated by a hint of medicine but their hearts will never be regulated by a hint of medicine and their lives are ragged and tattered and bent in ways that make you insane with rage when you think about it too long.

*

Consider the long and intricate and colorful history of the study of the heart. The first cardiac surgeons were certainly practicing long before recorded history. Imagine how many hearts were cut from the chests of enemies and slaves and sacrificial victims and eaten, burned, buried, mounted as trophies, thrown disdainfully to the clamoring dogs. But with howling savagery comes relentless curiosity, that being the human way, blood and brilliance together, and soon enough came the Roman doctor Claudius Galen, who attended to emperors and gladiators, and wrote detailed works on the anatomy and physiology of the heart; and the Italian doctor Realdo Columbo, who figured out how pulmonary circulation and heart valves really worked; and the hotheaded English doctor William Harvey, son of the mayor of Folkestone, who saw finally the simple brilliance of the circulatory system and explained it to a world he knew would be infuriated by the disproving of centuries-old belief:

"I dread lest I have all men as enemies," wrote Harvey, after he published his discoveries, "so much does reverence for ambiguity influence all men. But now the die is cast; my hope is in the love of truth and the integrity of intelligence."

What faith in the love of truth and the integrity of intelligence! So: was William Harvey right to have faith in the ultimate grace of his fellow beings, or was he a dolt?

*

Or the Swedish doctor Olof Rudbeck the Elder, the woodcarver who opened eels and fish and cats and dogs and felt their beating hearts with his finger to trace their blood flow; or the Cornish doctor Richard Lower, who discovered that blood "could be transferred outside the confine of its own body for the health of a second" person; or the Florentine doctor Lorenzo Bellini, who discovered that coronary arteries could clog unto death; or the Roman doctor Giovanni Maria Lancisi, who first described heart attacks ("internal pains of the chest, accompanied at one moment by difficulty of breathing, especially when ascending hills, and at another by a strangling sensation of the heart and frequently by an uneven pulse"); or the Copenhagen doctor Niels Stensen, who looked and looked for the magic innate spirit and soul and vitality inside the heart, the secret chamber from which issued the essence of character and personality, and finally concluded, politely, in a book he wrote in 1664, at the age of twenty-six, that there was no such thing: "The heart has been considered the seat of natural warmth, as the throne of the soul, and even as the soul itself. Some have greeted the heart as the sun, others as the king; but if you examine it more closely, one finds it to be nothing more than a muscle."

A miraculous muscle, to be sure; but a muscle subject to entropy and failure, malfunction and malaise, storm and shatter.

*

Or the Croatian doctor Duro Armeno, also called Giorgio Baglivi, who discovered that the heart could beat independently of its contiguous body, which he discovered by cutting out frogs' hearts and leaving them to beat in the sunlight; or the Anglican priest Stephen Hales, first to measure venous and arterial blood pressure, which he did by slicing open the left carotid artery of an elderly mare one cold December day in 1714 in the village of Teddington in Middlesex and measuring the spurting blood of the dying horse, to which he had affixed the excised windpipe of a goose and a glass tube twelve feet high. The mare, in her last moments, shot her blood more than nine feet high in the tube when her heart contracted, the blood level falling as her heart relaxed, the pattern of highs and lows ebbing as she died.

The Reverend Stephen Hales is honored and celebrated today as a father of hemodynamics, the patron saint of the blood-pressure cuff we have all worn as the rhythm of our blood is measured, and by all accounts he was a sensitive and remarkable man who, as he wrote after the death of the mare, "did not then pursue the Matter any further, being discouraged by the Disagreeableness of Anatomic Dissection," and he devoted his later years to the study of circulation in plants, and he designed a water system for his village, and he designed ventilation systems for crowded English prisons and hospitals, and he co-founded the Royal Society of Arts and was instrumental in awarding grants to young artists, and he later was instrumental in figuring out that kidney stones

could be dissolved, and he is still so revered as a botanist that
there is a tree named for him (Halesia, or snowdrop tree) and
the American Society of Plant Physiologists annually presents
the Stephen Hales Award for outstanding contributions to the
field; but that cold December day stays with me, the elderly
mare "which was otherwise to be killed as unfit for service,"
the moist ground, the cawing ravens, the brass cannula in
Hales' hand as he reaches into the heart of the horse, the wild
eye of the horse, the grim look on the face of the stablehand
as he sits on the horse's head, the leap of blood in the glass
tube, the way Hales kneels and caresses the horse's jaw and
she looks at him and he looks at her and what she is really, the
horseness of her, the equine essence, her sweet salty spirit that
never was before and will never be again, flies away.

*

Or the Bolognese doctor Giovanni Battista Morgagni,
who suggested that doctors should listen to "the cry of the
suffering organs," and invented the idea that diseases of the
heart could be understood by physical analysis of the failed
heart in autopsy (and who with his wife Paola had fifteen
children, eight of whom became nuns, and one a priest); or
the French doctor Jean-Baptiste de Senac, the first to prescribe
quinine for "long and rebellious palpitations" of the heart;
or the Swiss doctor Albrecht von Haller, who confirmed that
animal hearts continued to beat even after removal from the
body (and who, perhaps racked with some dark guilt after
removing so many living hearts from living creatures, became
addicted to opiates in his last years); or the Scottish doctor
John Hunter, who wrote books on the Natural History of the
Human Teeth and on Gun-Shot Wounds, and whose prime
heart patient was himself, as his clogged heart failed him in
his old age; he noted, with dour perspicacity, that his attacks

of angina pectoris were brought on not only by exertion but by high emotion: "My life is at the mercy of any rogue who chooses to provoke me," he said, shortly before he lost his temper during a hospital board meeting and ran gasping from the room and died in the arms of a friend.

*

Or the man for whom the word *volt* is named, Alessandro Volta of Como, called *il mago benefico* by his neighbors, the good magician, who was born, as he said, poorer than poor on the shores of Lake Como, and did not speak for four years, his first word being, as all readers with children will guess, a vehement *no!*, but eventually he spoke six languages fluently, and would become so absorbed by a problem that he would not eat or sleep for days at a time, especially when riveted by electrical matters, which fascinated him utterly, including such electrical matters as the passage of electricity through muscle, which is what happens inside the heart, which is an astounding muscle lit and livid with electricity. *Il mago benefico* invented the battery, and the electroscope, among many other contraptions and magic machines, but as much as I love batteries, and the way Volta's work laid the groundwork for the electrical ingenuity that allows me to type these words and see what I am typing and not be shivering in the cold spring rain, I am most grateful to the man from Como for the way he built the floor for cardiac electrophysiology and electrocardiography, which are cool long words for the way there is a divine pulse in the heart.

*

So many brilliant students of the heart, all over the world, so many shy intrepid explorers of the new countries of the heart: the Gloucestershire doctor Edward Jenner, who discovered that coronary arteries could clog and choke the heart they fed, and the Irish doctor Dominic Corrigan, who studied the dissonant musics of flawed hearts, their murmurs and rumbles and thrills and bruits, and the Breton surgeon Rene Laennec, who invented the stethoscope, and the Dutch doctor Frans Donders, first to actually record the sounds of the heart, and the Polish doctor Wilhelm Ebstein, who invented the idea (in 1898!) that a low-carbohydrate diet was good for the heart, and the German doctor Friedrich Maass, who invented cardiopulmonary resuscitation by saving a nine-year-old boy named Heinrich who had been accounted dead, and the Canadian doctor Maude Abbott, who loved nothing better than a party, and the Welsh cardiologist Thomas Lewis, who studied the effect of war on soldiers' hearts, and the British doctor George Mines, who was so interested in dysrhythmia in the heart that he induced it in himself and was found dead in his laboratory at age twenty-nine, and the great Mexican surgeon Ignacio Chavez and the great Cuban surgeon Agustin Castellanos, and The Mother of Pediatric Cardiology, the American doctor Helen Brooke Taussig, who was stone deaf and dyslexic, the renowned American transplant surgeon Michael DeBakey from Louisiana, who sewed Dacron grafts on a sewing machine before putting them in his patients, or the Slovakian doctor William Ganz, who survived Auschwitz, or the South African surgeon Christiaan Barnard, who did the first heart transplant ever but had to retire young because of savage arthritis, or the former University of Texas basketball star Denton Cooley, who did, wrote Barnard, "the most beautiful surgeries I have ever seen," and Brian Barratt-Boyes of New Zealand and Chuichi Kawai of Japan and Pavlos Toutouzas of Greece and and and …

So many hands on hearts, hands in hearts, heads on hearts. All over the world, for thousands of years, men and women exploring and healing the wet engine.

3. Hope

Dave's mom is named Hope. She is seventy-nine years old. She was born on Post Street in San Francisco. Her mother was a nurse. Her father grew flowers. When she was an infant her father was crushed by a train. When she was seven her brother drowned in the bay. When she was seventeen she and her mother and brother and sister were evicted from their home by order of the federal government of the United States and sent to live in a horse stall at a racetrack with other men and women and children of Japanese ancestry.

My brother slept in the front of the stall, she says, and my mother and sister and I slept in the rear of the stall. It was raining on the night we arrived there. We were given Army mattress covers and told to go to the barn and fill them with hay. We were there six months. Then we were sent to Camp Topaz in Utah. It was in the high desert. The barracks were made of wood and tar paper. In the winter it was very cold and in the summer the dust came through the windows and doors and walls.

In the camp I went to high school and became engaged to a boy named Hiroshi. His family was ordered to Japan on prisoner exchange. I went with them. We were two months at sea. We slept on the deck. We washed our hair in the rain when the rain came every afternoon. We went around Africa. The captain of the ship told us one day that Japan was losing the war and there wasn't enough food in Japan and he would let us off the ship before we got to Japan if we wanted to get off. All the young people on the ship had a meeting and we decided to get off the ship in Singapore or Manila. I got off in Singapore. All the ones who got off in Manila died. Where I was the bombs fell all around. When the war ended all I had was the clothes on my back. Many ladies were scared of rape so they cut their hair real short like a man. I did not.

I went on to Japan. First time I ever set foot there. It was very cold and we sewed coats and pants from blankets. I left Hiroshi because he treated me badly. I found a job with the United States Eighth Army. That's how I met my husband. His name was Art. He had red hair. He was Scottish, English, Irish, and Cherokee was in there too. All the other American soldiers worked very hard but he seemed to spend all his time fooling around and teasing the girls. One day the promotion list came out and I took his name off. He didn't get the promotion. When he found out he came storming into the office and read me up and down and I heard words I never heard before. Two weeks later he came to apologize and he brought me silk stockings. A month later he invited me to the theater with him. We went to see the *Mikado*. That was our first date.

After a while he asked me to get married. I said no: I had to go home and find out what happened to my family. So he said okay, fine, and he went home to Oklahoma. A year later I went home and when my ship came into San Francisco there was Art waiting for me at the wharf. He asked me to get married again and I said no again. He went to my family and asked my brother if he could marry me and my brother said no. I went to work at a hospital and lived in a rooming house, and Art was working for the railroad and living in another rooming house, and he kept asking me to get married and I kept saying no but finally one day I said yes. We got married in the morning at city hall and moved in together that afternoon and I was so excited I got sick, and that was our honeymoon, me sick in our new apartment and Art taking care of me.

Hope folds her hands in her lap and smiles. She tells me about their two sons, one named for Davy Crockett, and about the house they built in the California mountains, and how her husband lost his voice at the end of his life, which was a great blow to the both of them, for he loved to tease her and she loved to hear him, and how when she was a little girl she loved to run barefoot in the city, and how in summer she and her sister and cousins and friends would sing on the roof of their building at night, huddled and hungry and happy, a long time ago but not very long ago at all.

*

Hope and her family were evicted from their home in 1942 by provision of Executive Order 9066, issued by Franklin Delano Roosevelt on February 19, 1942. "Whereas the successful prosecution of the war requires every possible protection against espionage and against sabotage," wrote FDR, "I hereby authorize and direct the Secretary of War to prescribe regulations for the conduct and control of alien enemies …"

One of which alien enemies was the shy teenage American girl Hope.

More than 110,000 American citizens of Japanese ancestry were eventually held in ten internment camps (or "concentration camps," as FDR himself called them) in the American West for the next two years. In March of 1942, Public Proclamation Number One created Military Areas Numbers One and Two, which comprised California, Oregon, Washington, and Arizona, the states from which the Nisei—Americans of Japanese heritage—would soon be excluded as possible alien enemies. Two weeks later Roosevelt established the War Relocation Authority, which carried out the task.

Amache, Colorado.

Gila River, Arizona.

Minidoka, Idaho.

Jerome, Arkansas.

Manzanar, California.

Heart Mountain, Wyoming.

Poston, Arizona.

Rohwer, Arkansas.

Tule Lake, California.

Topaz, Utah.

One hundred and ten thousand children and women and men.

Evacuees, the government called these of its citizens.

Prisoners, inmates, internees, they call themselves.

How do we count them?

As the late Oregon poet William Stafford said:

One.

One.

One …

*

O Topaz, o one square mile of wind and dust, o searing light and wrenching cold, with your forty-two blocks each exactly the same, each grid with thirteen barrack buildings and a recreation hall and a mess hall and a laundry and a pile of coal and a latrine and shower stalls and a manager's office and one tree. The Paiute Indians who had lived there for centuries immemorial called it Pahvant, the place of abundant water, which it was before white settlers diverted the Sevier River for irrigation and made it what the first white American maps called it: the Sevier Desert, on which only greasewood and saltgrass grew. And forty-two trees—elms, olives, junipers, and locusts, sent by the forestry department at Utah State College, which also sent ten thousand cuttings of tamarisk and willows and currants. Which all soon died in the heat and wind and salt soil.

Rank on rank the forty-two blocks were stacked around the center of camp, where were the schools and libraries and churches and post office and gymnasium. To the north, administrative offices, the hospital, the military police station; to the south a fifteen-acre community garden plot, playing fields (of raked dust), and the cemetery that was never used for the 144 prisoners who died during the life of the camp; their bodies were sent to Salt Lake City for cremation and their ashes held for their families to claim after the war.

Around the perimeter of camp, every inch of it, a tall barbed wire fence. Around the perimeter, every quarter mile, watchtowers with searchlights and armed guards. Pinned to the lapels of the prisoners arriving at Topaz: identification tags.

The first two hundred prisoners arrived, by train, on September 11, 1942. Then five hundred prisoners on September 16. Then five hundred prisoners a day until October 16. All told more than eight thousand prisoners in five weeks.

Each contingent of prisoners greeted by a drum and bugle corps at the front gate.

Among the prisoners: Shirley Temple's gardener.

*

On June 25, 1943, the first graduation class in Topaz High School history conducted its commencement exercises on the plaza in front of the high school building. It was windy. It was always windy, says Hope.

The graduating class entered the plaza to the strains of the English hymn "Jerusalem," based on a poem by the mystic genius William Blake. After the Pledge of Allegiance, and the playing of the American national anthem, and a prayer led by a Protestant minister, Mr. Joseph Tsukamoto, and songs by the German composers Johann Sebastian Bach and Richard Wagner and the Polish composer Frederic Chopin, there was a flurry of speeches, and translation of them into Japanese by graduating senior Motoichi Yanagi, and presentation of the 216 degrees, and then the class sang the alma mater (… *from far and wide we've gathered, and made now into one* …), and then the choir sang "Jerusalem" again and marched off to a reception in Dining Hall No. 32. So ended the first year of Topaz High School in Topaz Internment Camp, Utah.

Soon thereafter the 1943 yearbook was published. *Ramblings*, it was called–the school's mascot being a ram–and along with its accounts of the doings of the dance committee and the newspaper staff and the thespian club and the choir and the Future Farmers of America chapter and the home economics club and the basketball team, there are pages and pages of photographs of and notes on the seniors, one of whom was Hope, and I spend hours and hours in these pages, staring at her face, and all the faces, and the yearning and grace and earnestness of these children break my heart.

Teruko wants to be a beautician. Minoru wants to be a surveyor. Stanley wants to be an entomologist. Mitsuyo wants to be a seamstress. Kazuko wants to be a dietician. Hisako wants to be a stenographer. Teiko wants to study mathematics. Kazuyuki wants to be a carpenter. Seiji wants to join the United States Army. Mariko wants to be a pharmacist. Hisashi wants to be a chef. Peter wants to be a farmer. Kazuo wants to be a mechanic. Masaru wants to be a writer. Umeko wants to be a housewife. Tomi says he wants to be the ideal husband.

Motoko wants to be an oculist. Minoru wants to be an actor. Miyeko wants to be a librarian. Eiji wants to be a chemical engineer. Fusaye wants to sing. Himeo wants to be the fastest runner ever. Yemiko wants to be a nurse. Rey wants to be an artist. Teruko wants to be a teacher. Okiko is looking forward to the day when she will become, as she says, a doctor.

Their faces peer at me from 1943, smiling, grinning, shy, scared, startled by the camera, their eyeglasses slightly askew, neckties neatly knotted, hair curled just so, stern, beaming, one boy wearing a rakish cap, one girl with a handkerchief meticulously folded into her blazer pocket. Hope's smile is big and confident.

After each senior's name and before each senior's feats and accomplishments and desires and dreams and ambitions and hopes and plans there is, in parentheses, the name of the high school he or she was attending before being sent to Camp Topaz. Oakland High, Berkeley High, San Mateo High, Alameda, Hayward, San Leandro, San Jose, Pescadero. Hilo and Konawaena in Hawaii. Pascal High in Texas. Theodore Roosevelt High School in Fresno. George Washington High in San Francisco.

*

On December 18, 1944, as Douglas MacArthur's soldiers and sailors and airmen and divers and intelligence agents drove through the Pacific theater toward Manila, their hearts and fears on the inevitable invasion of Japan, the United States War Relocation Authority announced plans to close all ten American concentration camps within six to twelve months. On August 6, 1945, the United States dropped an atomic bomb on Hiroshima. The Americans called the bomb Little Boy and the Japanese called it the Original Child. The fireball created by the bomb was one hundred million degrees at its center and burned one hundred and thirty thousand people to death by the end of the day. On August 9 the United States dropped an atomic bomb on Nagasaki. Seventy-five thousand people burned to death by the end of the day. On August 14 Japan surrendered. On August 15 the first prisoners were released from Topaz, heading back to the Pacific coast. On September 2 the war was formally ended by signature in Tokyo Bay. Hope's family went home to San Francisco. On October 31, at one in the afternoon, the camp's front gate was locked from the outside after the last prisoners were released—mostly families from Hawaii waiting for space on ships to get home.

In three years at Topaz there had been two assaults, two major thefts, six arrests for public drunkenness, ten arrests for gambling, thirteen prisoners sent to mental hospitals, eighteen prisoners sent to Japan, one hundred and seventy-eight prisoners joining the United States Army, one hundred and thirty-nine deaths, and three hundred and eight-four births.

Topaz's nineteen thousand acres was eventually sold (for a dollar an acre) to local farmers, who also bought many of the buildings to use as chicken coops and tool sheds. By 1966 nothing remained of the camp but concrete barrack foundations and a laundry boiler smokestack.

In 1976 the Japanese American Citizen League of Salt Lake City bought an acre of camp land (near what had been the front gate) and erected a commemorative marker.

In 1988 the President of the United States, Ronald Reagan, signed House Resolution 442 into law, directing the government to issue a formal apology and pay $20,000 to each surviving prisoner.

In 1990 the first payments were actually issued, accompanied by a letter from the President of the United

States: "We can never fully right the wrongs of the past," wrote George Bush the elder, "but we can take a clear stand for justice and recognize that serious injustices were done to Japanese Americans during World War II."

In 1993 a newly constituted Topaz Museum committee bought most of the campsite back (for fifty dollars an acre) and, working with the Utah State Historical Society, began to restore the camp. So far there's half a building standing amid the greasewood and saltgrass—half an old pine-and-tar camp recreation hall, through which the wind whistles freely, blazing in summer and frigid in winter.

I ask Hope if she remembers the recreation hall. O yes, she says. Yes. I remember the wind and the dust coming through the windows. It was always so windy in camp. You could not escape that wind. It would find you. It lived with you.

I ask her if she is bitter about being imprisoned by her own government for having parents from another country.

No, I am not bitter, she says. No. Bitter is no place to be. But I do not forget.

4. Imo Pectore

Unto me and my wife one day two sons are born, a minute apart. Two boys lifted mewling from the salt sea of her uterus: one darkhaired, one light; one small, one large; one with a healthy heart, and the other,

Not.

*

Heartache, heartsore, heartsick, heartbroken. My heart is hammered. My heart moans. My heart is splintered and ragged and shattered and shuttered. My heart is cold. My heart is heavy. My heart is hard. My heart is a stone, flint, iron, a fist.

We knew that one of the babies would have a flawed heart, according to sonograms taken while they were in utero, and we'd been told that it was likely that that one would have to have surgery right away, but we hoped against hope that it wouldn't be so.

But it is so.

I wake my wife and tell her. Her eyes go gray.

*

We give the boys names to carry all their lives: the small darkhaired darkeyed one, the fox-boy, a tiny coyote, a child the size and color of mink, his eyes wide, his attention laser, this lean droplet of boy lifted from his mother's torn belly, this one, the firstborn, is given the name Joseph, an ancient sturdy name, from the Greek Iosephos, from the Hebrew Yoseph, meaning: *God adds him to the world*. The name worn by the brawny muscled silent stepfather of the Christos.

And the second boy, the lighthaired cheerful round large one, with a chamber missing from his heart: his name takes a while to arrive, which worries us, because it seems bad luck to leave him nameless, especially with knives hanging over his heart, but we had only agreed on his name if he was a girl, which he isn't, so he cannot be Gina, so my wife suggests Henry, and I suggest Liam, and we mull this over for a while, and then sleepily she says *Liam*, and so he is given the name Liam, an ancient Irish name, thought to have meant helmet or protection before the English came to Ireland and savaged that green rocky world and so many of its green liquid words.

I whisper his new name into the boy's ear, whisper a prayer that it will protect him from pain, that it will be a helmet of a name, for he will always be at war, he will always be wounded, he is wounded right from the first minute he enters this bruised broken blessed world.

*

The days pass one by one and the doctors watch the second boy with sharp eyes and they say every day no, no surgery yet, no, wait and watch, no, there's a hole in his heart that if it closes we will do the surgery immediately, but if it doesn't close there's no immediate hurry, and it doesn't close, day after day, and every day the sweet quiet nurses help my wife as she tries to nurse her two new sons, the dark jittery first one who cries every time he is removed from the warm country of her chest and the light calm second one who is accompanied always by a web and thicket of tubes and wires and sensors, and the hole in the calm one's heart doesn't close and doesn't close and finally after a week we are all sent home, my wife and our two new roommates.

*

A week later we meet Dave for the first time. He's in his green scrubs. He crouches down again and again and draws for my wife and me the architecture of Liam's heart, and she and I pay ferocious attention together so our two brains will maybe together understand what Dave is saying, and he says *Liam's heart is perfectly balanced physiologically with the right amount of pulmonary blood flow,* and he explains about fenestration and pressure, and valvular function and oxygenation and malfunction, and he has a blue pen and a red pen and he charts flow and flaw, he shows us where the surgeon will eventually build a shunt, and reroute veins, and we watch absorbed, with complete and furious attention, we *must* understand, but I understand nearly nothing, for the veins and arteries swirl and whip before my eyes as Dave draws, and I am swirling and lost, so scared I can hardly speak. He draws and draws, his patience oceanic, and then he is called away, and he stands up with the quick sure motion of a cat and he vanishes in a green blur and we sit there with his drawings in our hands, staring at blue rivers and red rivers.

*

Imagine Dave squatting in front of you. He's in his green scrubs. You and your wife are perched on the edge of your chairs looking into his eyes and staring at the sheets of paper in his hands. You remember every word that comes out of his mouth because every word is your son, your son's life, your son's heart, your fear, your love.

Single ventricle, says Dave. Usually there are two, right and left. In his case his heart is actually flipped over as well.

Unusual. It's a good thing for him. Gives us better access.

Access, I think. Access to his *heart*. Access for scalpels and electrodes and the fingers of surgeons. His heart will be *open to the air*.

Complex congenital cyanotic heart disease, says Dave. Situs solitus of the viscera, ventricular inversion with hypoplasia of the right ventricle and tricuspid valve, ventriculoarterial discordance, annular pulmonary and subvalvular stenosis. Essentially intact atrial septum, though. That's good.

Pause.

Dave?

Okay, says Dave. What this means is that he only has one ventricle and he needs two; we can't build him a second one because of the shape and formation of his heart; his heart is reversed from the usual orientation; but he has *beautiful* anatomy for what we need to do. What we need to do is called a Fontan procedure. We're pretty sure that's the only way to go. It's a two-stage operation. The first would be when he's two or three months old and the second when he's between eighteen and thirty months.

Two heart operations?

Yes.

And if they succeed?

Then he has a heart and venous system that should carry him to and probably past puberty.

After which?

Transplant. Or whatever we've invented by then.

What if the operations don't work?

Liam is a very good candidate for the Fontan, says Dave. He's a vigorous baby. His color is excellent. He has adequate fat stores. *Beautiful* anatomy. All the signs are good. He should do very well.

What if he doesn't?
He should do very well.

*

When the pope makes a decision about the naming of a
cardinal, but declines to name that new cardinal publicly,
because to name him publicly would bring unwelcome
attention, which is to say that the government or regime or
junta or dictatorship or commissariat or executive committee
of the nation in which the new cardinal resides would be even
more interested than usual in stilling the heart of the new
cardinal, for fear of his increased influence on the hearts of the
faithful in his country, then the pope keeps the new cardinal's
name *imo pectore*–in the innermost recess of his heart. Other
than His Holiness the Pontiff of Rome, no one knows how
many more cardinals there are in the world than we think
there are. Their names are revealed only after they die. Many
times in the long history of the Holy Roman Catholic Church
the Pope has died suddenly without having the chance to
inform anyone of the cardinals he holds in his heart; so when
that particular pope's heart ceased to beat, the names of his
secret cardinals flew from their muscular home and vanished.
The more I think about this the more riveting it is to me.
Lesson: there are secret words in every heart. For almost ten
years now I have had five secret words in the innermost recess
of my heart, and I reach in there sometimes and unpack the
box they're in and inhale their redolent spice, always fresh,
always restorative, always miraculous water to a thirsty man:
he should do very well. I don't forget those words. Those are
good words.

*

At four months of age Liam had a cardiac catheterization–a procedure during which the anesthesiologist knocked him out cold with chloral hydrate (the drug that, combined with alcohol, composes the knockout drops, the Mickey Finns, of pulp literature), Dave made an incision in his left groin, ran a catheter tube into his heart through his left femoral vein, and looked around inside his tiny heart. Once during the procedure Liam's heart fluttered and once it raced madly for sixty seconds; Dave calmed the flutter with a jolt of electricity and regulated the racing with a shot of atropine, a drug extracted from the plant called, darkly, nightshade.

A week later I went to the blood bank and pumped out a pint of A-positive for my son, my heart shoving it out of me into a bag from which it would be eventually pumped into Liam's heart.

At five months of age Liam had a median sternotomy, an atrial septecomy, and a bi-directional Glenn procedure. Or: his chest, no bigger than my hand, was cut open, his chestbone halved with bone shears, and the blood vessels north of his heart rearranged variously, one sewn to another, one throttled with a rubber band.

Why did they do that to Liam? asked his sister Lily, three years old.

To fix his heart.

Is it fixed?

Half way.

Will they fix it all the way?

Yes.

When?

Next year.

Will he stay alive until then?

Yes.

Are you sure or should I ask Mom?

I'm sure.

*

The Fontan procedure is named for Francis Maurice Fontan, who is now seventy-six years old, lives in Bordeaux, works and teaches at the University of Bordeaux and at the Clinique Saint-Augustin, speaks beautiful English, retired three years ago from active surgery, enjoys opera and golf, and is the creative genius who, thirty years ago, invented a new way of surgically dealing with the lack of a functioning pumping chamber in the hearts of new children with complex heart disease.

What if, *le docteur* Fontan proposed, blood returning to the heart from the body could be channeled to the lungs in a *passive* fashion, without the pumping chamber? Or: what if the surgeon connected the veins carrying blood returning from the body (the vena cavae) directly to the vessels carrying blood to the lungs (the pulmonary arteries)? The blood would be reoxygenated, the missing chamber wouldn't be a problem, and the generally relentless mobility of the human body–the fact that in the normal course of their daily lives people move around a lot, sitting, standing, walking, kneeling, bending, crouching, running, dancing, gesticulating, stomping, leaping, cursing, singing, shouting, weeping, howling, laughing—would ensure continual flow, if not at the ideally regulated pressure of pumped blood. Essentially, Fontan reasoned, circulation patterns akin to normal would be created in patients with hearts that were not normal.

"We cardiac surgeons," Doctor Fontan writes to me from Bordeaux, "already had the experience of the superior vena cava to right pulmonary artery derivation, invented experimentally by an Italian surgeon, and performed in human beings for the first time by a Russian surgeon, and popularized in Western medical literature by an American surgeon. The Russian surgeon had published his findings in Russian medical literature, but his works were totally ignored for years by the rest of the world; it was the time of the Cold War and of the Iron Curtain. So, I said to myself, what works for superior vena cava to right pulmonary artery derivation should probably work as well for inferior vena cava to left pulmonary artery derivation; and this was the case."

*

And this was the case! So gently said, so taut a phrase, so precise, just the five words, a little quitrain, a cincosyllabic poem sung by the French gentleman, another little five-word boat sailing across my heart; but o the lives changed by those five words, boys and girls and men and women, in every nation, in villages and towns and cities from sea to sea and pole to pole ...

*

"I performed the first Fontan myself," continues *le docteur,* "in April of 1968. I reported our first cases in the literature only in 1971, because I wanted to be sure that the results of the operation were durable before attracting colleagues to a dead end."

The Fontan procedure *was* "durable," it turned out— but difficult to accomplish surgically, given the tiny size and immense complexity of infant and toddler hearts. And cardiologists soon discovered that Fontan procedures also sometimes had unusual attendant consequences, among them post-operative fluid leakage in the chest cavity and a diminution of efficient food processing. The sixty percent of patients who survive Fontan procedures are at much higher risk than normal for arrhythmias, blood vessel deterioration, blood clots, protein-losing enteropathy, edema, pleural and pericardial effusions, and many other ills large and small.

Or: many small Fontan patients, for all sorts of reasons, die.

*

But Liam didn't die. He spent the year after the first stage of his Fontan operation guzzling milk from his mama and belching like a barge and learning to sit up and developing a face as round as a planet and developing a ferocious yen for cheerios and pears and learning to stand up and walk around the room holding on to couches and chairs and tables and people and then learning to sail off on his own waddling and shuffling and then walking and then running here and there and occasionally smacking his face on something or other and occasionally smacking his twin brother and once or twice his older sister although he quickly proved his intelligence by grokking the fact that she was stronger and meaner and quicker when it came to blows rained down upon the boys who were suddenly crowding her existence which heretofore had been filled with fawning parents and now appeared to be filled with Chaos and Hubbub, which is what her father called her brothers so often that occasionally visitors were under the temporary impression that indeed such vaguely Hebraic names had been inflicted upon the squirming boychiks.

That was a good time, what I remember of it. I remember changing a lot of diapers and laughing a lot and not sleeping very much. That was a good time.

*

"When a patient dies," the piercingly honest Doctor Fontan writes me, "we surgeons cannot ourselves offer more than some degree of sadness for the patient and compassion for the family, otherwise we would not survive intellectually and emotionally. I have two colleagues who had to stop operating on patients altogether because they were too much affected when their patients died.

"But, you know, most of your patients live, and you have helped them live. That is good knowledge. Many of my Fontan patients keep in touch with me. I see them becoming teenagers, adults, enter professions, get married, have children, which is really something special for my female Fontan patients, because of course pregnancy and birth strain the heart very much."

I imagine Doctor Fontan at the wedding of one of his patients. She is, let us say, a willowy young lady—Fontan patients, for some reason no one understands, tend to grow tall and lean. Let us call her Veronique. She is, let us say, twenty-five years old. She is a striking young woman with an aura of calm energy; a verb of a woman. Doctor Fontan operated on her when she was six months old and then again when she was eighteen months old. He does not of course remember those operations specifically, as they were a long time ago and she was an infant and then a toddler and surgeons tend to think of their patients as problems to be solved rather than as personalities. Yet something about the Veroniqueness of Veronique stayed with him, something snagged his heart, her zest and verve and humor and dogged courage, perhaps; and he has made a point, let us say, of never missing her annual checkup, and annually it gives him pleasure to shake her hand and note her progress, and she has presented him one or two of the bright watercolors she has begun to paint, and he has presented her with a copy of his favorite novel by Marguerite Yourcenar, *Memoirs of Hadrian*, because Veronique mentioned that she wishes someday to write a novel, and so, last year, when she presented him with an engraved invitation to her wedding, he was honored and delighted, and accepted on the spot, and today, the morning of the wedding, he is one of the first people to the chapel, and he finds a seat in the tiny balcony, from which he watches the whole brave theatrical ancient holy parade of the ceremony, during which, to his surprise, he finds himself much moved, and contemplating the fact that once, a long time ago, he held this child's beating heart in his hand, and made of that flawed moist machine a thing healthy enough for her to hand to a lover.

*

When Liam was sixteen months old Dave had him knocked out again and peered into his heart, this time with two catheters, both snaking up through his groin into his heart. Dave kept up a running monologue during the procedure, which was recorded. So here's Dave talking to himself during the catheterization: "Yes, right ventricle appears to be half the volume of the left ventricle … we can see enlarged left ventricle … Liam thankfully has very nice pulmonary arteries … some volume overload to his single ventricle anatomy … in all likelihood he will be a very satisfactory candidate for completion of his Fontan …"

Which was completed two months later. Again the anesthesia, again the bone shears, again the ice on his heart, again the cutting and stitching, again the tape over his eyes so he would not see and startle at the bright lights and masked faces, again the massive drugs, again his parents huddled in the shadowy waiting room, again family and friends milling gently through the days and nights, again Dave crouching before us with his gentle intent grin and his hands drawing red lines and blue lines on the charts of the heart, again Liam emerging from the dark and blinking and moaning. Five days later Dave says Liam is well enough to go home and he writes Liam a pass out of the hospital. My wife Mary dresses her bruised boy and puts him gently in his stroller with his bear and wheels boy and bear through the corridors and hallways and elevators. As they near the front doors of the hospital Liam gets all restless and fussy and fidgety and causes a ruckus. Mary, as perceptive a woman as there ever was, realizes what he wants and lifts him out of the stroller and he swaggers through the swinging front doors of the hospital himself.

Once through the doors he tires and Mary hoists him back into the stroller and we take him home.

Eight years later I remember the way I felt deep in my hoary heart that day when he pushed through those big doors, curious, delighted, hard-headed, sore-hearted, hungry for light. I like to tell him that story and he likes to hear it, about the time he was one tough hombre even though he was only one and one half year old, and he met pain head-on and kicked its butt and told that pain he would *remember* its ugly face and if ever pain troubled his town again, why, there would be some hell raised and some thrashin' and bashin', you hear that, you ugly pain?, and sometimes if he is feeling especially goofy and showoffy and nutty he will imitate his own swagger that day, and every time this happens, which happens about once a year or so, I get a feeling in my chest that there aren't enough words for.

*

"I was myself attracted by pediatric cardiac surgery," says Doctor Fontan, "because in the late 1950s, when I was a young trainee in surgery, the field of congenital cardiac malformations was the most attractive intellectually and the most demanding surgically, a field where almost everything was to be discovered and where firm operative procedures had to be established."

I tell Dave about this remark one day, and he says yeh, isn't it amazing that a few short years ago an awful lot of pediatric heart patients would just die, and now they don't? And I say yeh, Dave, that's amazing, and then a few hours later when I am doing the dishes I suddenly think, you know, *amazing* just isn't a big enough word for the fact that thousands of kids don't die now.

*

In the nine years since Liam survived the operation that Francis Fontan invented, my son has been a Normal Boy, which is to say, in his particular case, that he has learned to use bad language, doesn't make his bed, reads avidly, has fought back against bullies in the playground, broke his shoulder-blade twice, loves ice cream and hamburgers, has become a fanatic San Antonio Spurs fan, prefers his skateboard to his bicycle, calls his sister names, prefers boxers to briefs, prefers rice to potatoes, never takes his Spurs hat off except for bed and shower, tells me his dreams, likes to read under the covers with a flashlight, and has read all eleven of the Lemony Snicket *Series of Unfortunate Events* novels in order, which is pretty impressive for a kid nine years old, I think—I mean, when I was nine, I was busy reading Silver Surfer comics.

Every year he goes to Dave for a thorough checkup and Dave looks under his hood. Over the years Dave has noticed that Liam bruises easily, is taller and thinner than his twin brother, tires noticeably after twenty minutes of vigorous exercise, has a slight mitral valve leak, and eventually will need a heart transplant, "though I hope that is decades away," says Dave.

Every year when Liam gets his checkup we sit and talk to Dave for a few minutes after the echocardiogram, and every year the transplant slides further away. A few years ago it was going to be right before Liam hit puberty, because puberty puts a terrific strain on the heart. Then it was going to be maybe age seventeen or so, when, as a surgeon told me bluntly, there are more teenage male hearts available because teenage boys die at a fairly high rate in car crashes. Then maybe the transplant would be at age twenty. Then thirty. Then forty. No one knows.

*

As I write these lines I look up and see Liam sprinting by, roaring, covered with mud and jelly. There's something about that boy, as my wife says, something calm, a grace mature far beyond his years; and while he can be the biggest rockhead ever born, and he runs like a old truck missing a wheel, and I have cleaned up far too many wedges of toast far-flung in petulance, I too have noticed an eerie grace in him, as if he is able to draw on a reserve tank of the stuff that most people can't summon. He calms people, I notice. He doesn't start fights, and although he's perfectly willing to poke his brother in the eye or pull his sister's hair when provoked, generally he breaks up fights, he defuses tension. Part of his charm is natural to any child but he seems to have a second gear that he brings to bear when needed; a grace suitable to need.

When he was born, with his missing chamber, and we thought he might die any day, I loved him inarticulately, and raged at his maker for making a broken boy, and many a night I sat rocking with him and thought about grace; what grace was this, to build a big pink boy with the bright face of an apple and a heart too weak to drive him through boyhood? A cruel gift of life and death at once. Now he is repaired for a while, a few years, a boyhood, before he needs a man's heart, and I have learned to shut my mouth and learn about grace: the deft grace of the doctors who edited him, the open grace of the thousand people who prayed for him in churches and temples and stupas and chapels and meeting houses, the grace with which he carries the body God gave him and Dave edited and surgeons carved in a way dreamed up by *le docteur* Francis Fontan.

I rub the peachfuzzcrewcutted head of my boy when he wanders past me in the kitchen, and I hold him in my arms when we sit on the couch in the dark marveling at ogres and orcs, and I rub his back at night, cupping his round face in my hand, whispering Gaelic in his ears, holding his hand when we cross streets, rubbing his legs and feet when he cries at night from growing pains, feeling his bicep when he flexes to show me he is more powerful than his many heroes, because there is always a jolt of joy in the touch, even when I am furious at him; because when I touch him *there he is,* and somehow my body never forgets the fear of the loss of his body. There's some kind of electric magnetic thing at play—an electric love in his heart and mine.

"Without touch, God is a monologue, an idea, a philosophy," wrote the late great American mystic Andre Dubus. "He must touch and be touched ... in the instant of the touch there is no place for thinking, for talking; the silent touch affirms all that, and goes deeper: it affirms the mysteries of love and mortality."

To which I say amen and then amen and then again amen.

5. Hagop

Dave McIrvin tells me a story, about a colleague of his named Hagop Hovaguimian. Hagop is fifty years old. He's a surgeon. He was born in Syria of Armenian descent. He's a genius, says Dave. The guy's unreal. He's a tremendous classical pianist and a tremendous surgeon and a tremendous skeet shooter. But he never plays the piano or shoots skeet or reads a book or goes out to dinner or takes a vacation or has a girlfriend. He just works. He doesn't do anything except work. He spends three months working with me and then he takes all the money he made over those three months and he goes to Armenia and pours it into the hospital he started there. He stays for nine months. Over there he lives in a little room in the hospital. I went with him once and stayed for a week and helped with operations. We completed operations by flashlight. We did operations where pencils were part of the surgical instrumentation. You wouldn't believe the conditions, the lack of electricity, the lack of amenities. An ancient broken torn lovely country. There are a million stories there. One time Hagop told me he had a patient who needed a kidney, a soldier, and one day another soldier showed up pushing a prisoner along, and the soldier says *this guy volunteered to donate a kidney to my buddy.* Hagop flags that, you know, but it turns out the prisoner *did* volunteer his kidney, in exchange for his freedom.

There are a lot of stories like that.

What Hagop has done there is incredible. He's saved so many lives. He's singlehandedly dragged his country toward modern medicine. Over there he's a hero. Over here he lives with his mother. Fascinating guy. Very quiet. Would never take any personal credit for what he's done. The only way he could be persuaded to talk to reporters about his hospital when he started it was because we convinced him that the more people who knew about the project the more people would help. Still, he was awfully uncomfortable. Fascinating guy. I've seen him drunk once in thirteen years. There was some event and somehow Hagop got into the brandy and like many people who hardly ever drink it was not a pretty sight. Turned out he thought he was a failure in life because he didn't join the army in Armenia and fight to defend his motherland. Can you believe it? A genius surgeon who has saved thousands of people in America and Armenia, and invented a hospital, I mean the guy *started his own hospital*, and he's thinking he's a failure because he wasn't a soldier *taking* lives.

People sure are complicated.

*

I talk to Hagop Hovaguimian one day, catching him between heart operations, a big one in the morning (boy, twenty months old) and two lesser ones in the afternoon (preemies, girls, each weighing two pounds). Hagop has eyes so dark they look obsidian. He's in his scrubs. His surgical mask is flopped open like a pale hand on his chest. His hair is waaay rumpled. He leans back in his chair in his office and talks quietly.

I was born in Aleppo, in Syria, he says. My parents were Armenian. I grew up there and went to med school there and did my residency there but then I wanted to be in the epicenter of medicine, where the textbooks were written, so I came to America. First I was in New York, doing general surgery, and then I came to Portland and learned cardiac surgery, and then I went to Philadelphia, to learn pediatric cardiac surgery, and then I came back to Portland to help start the pediatric cardiac program at this hospital, so now I have been here for a while.

My work in Armenia, that started with the collapse of the Soviet Union. A lot of people around the world felt optimistic when that happened. We felt that maybe the world's bipolar condition was finished. I felt a great optimism. Armenia was independent for the first time in a very long time. That was a great joy. But Armenia was in ruins. Yet I felt a new thing might be born there, so I decided to go see what could be done. I wanted to help build my motherland up again from the collapse of the empire. It was a romantic hopeful thing.

Well, I found that cardiac surgery there was frozen in the past. It was in the stone age. So I looked for equipment, and found just enough to get started. I came back to Oregon and made a team of people here and we went back to Armenia in the winter and we did fifteen heart operations on little children. We had no electricity or heat and we did operations by flashlight. I remember one kid who was brought in at six o'clock one night and he was going to die and we had no operating room. We found a room and put all our equipment in, tables and anesthesiology machine and heart/lung machine and everything, and so we made an operating room in about an hour, and we operated, and he survived.

He died a year later, that kid, but I will always remember making a room in a hurry in which to operate on him.

*

Dave came with me that time, says Hagop. He was one of the people I asked to be on the team. He said yes right away. I remember one night in Armenia we were tired and sitting. It was very cold and we were very tired. A family popped in with their half-dead baby who was severely cyanotic. Transposition of the great arteries with intact ventricular septum and patent ductus arteriosus. The solution is fairly simple; you essentially take the heart out, turn it around, and put it back in again.

A straightforward condition; without treatment the patient dies, with treatment the patient becomes normal. In America we would stabilize the child and then operate. But then, in Armenia, we had nothing. Dave and I looked each other. It was very cold. The computers in our heads were whirring, you know? We were thinking fast what could be done. But we had no equipment and there was nothing we could do. So in the morning the kid died. It's weird, you know? If you travel sixteen hours from where we sit right now you could be in a place where there is nothing you could do for a baby who is about to die. So.

*

Now, says Hagop, the Nork Marash Medical Center in Yerevan, which is the capital of Armenia, has nearly three hundred employees and we have saved 5,500 children. We've done every heart operation there is. We did 760 hearts last year, children and adults. One of the hearts that was repaired there five years ago was mine. I had a coronary bypass done there, by a surgeon I had trained. I was in my room in the hospital in the morning, washing my face, when I realized *I* was having a heart attack. So I walked down to the operating room.

*

I used to know the name of every kid who died, says Hagop. Not any more. There were too many. I don't remember the early years very well at all now. I remember the failures. I suppose I am suffering from the fact that my dream came true. Maybe I didn't dream big enough to keep me going. I don't play the piano much any more. I stopped feeling the need to play. But I love to do operations. I love the parents and families of the children. I love the sick people. This is love. It's an addiction for me, I think. Stress and reward. I love to be in the operating room with the music playing gently. For very difficult operations we play classical music. Baroque for the hardest of all. Bach or Vivaldi. Never the Romantics. You want to have it soothe and calm you but you don't want to have to pay close attention. So we never listen to Mozart or Beethoven. They are too commanding. And never opera. You couldn't operate to Puccini. For lesser cases we listen to soft rock. The Beatles, Elvis, Sting. The anesthesiologists are in charge of the music.

*

I'll tell you one last story about Dave, says Hagop. Did you know he brought a child back with us from that first trip to Armenia? A girl, thirteen years old, so sick she looked like she was six years old. We needed to have a heart/lung machine to be able to operate on her. There was something about her that just got to Dave. I asked him if he was sure about bringing her back to America and he was sure. When he's sure about something he's very sure. Well, we brought her back here, and found a place for her to stay, and found the money to pay for her operation, and took care of all the paperwork and everything, and we operated, and she survived, and we sent her back, and I saw her six years later, when she was nineteen, and she had just gotten married. So.

*

The phone rings and Hagop has to go do a patent ductus arteriosus operation on a child the size of his fist. I ask him one last question, about Dave, with whom he has worked now for thirteen years. He smiles.

I remember meeting Dave for the first time, says Hagop. He was such an energetic kid, so restless. And still all these years later no one enjoys what he is doing as much as Dave does. Also his mind is always beyond what he is doing daily. He has a deeper and further perspective than anyone. He is a most interesting man. He sees many things. A most restless man.

6. Joyas Volardores

Let us consider creatures great and small, green and blue, vegetative and mammalian, avian and human, all shells for all sorts of hearts. Let us begin with one particular shy elegant green silent creature, the foxglove plant, *Digitalis purpurea*. A common plant here in the Pacific Northwest; I see it nodding at me everywhere in late summer, taller than my children, leaning meditatively over the shoulders of highways, empurpling hillsides, standing watch over the dens and burrows of foxes and ground squirrels. An invader, native to Ireland but now spread everywhere in the New and Old Worlds. *Mearacan dearg* in the Gaelic. Produces a wide range of flowers in shades from white to pink to lavender. Pollinated mostly by bees: bumblebees, carpenter bees, honeybees, leafcutter bees, plaster bees, digger bees, mason bees, halictid bees. First named in formal herbology in 1542 by a German botanist and doctor named Leonard Fuchs, who called it *digitulus*, little finger, for the thimble shape of its flowers. Popularized as medicine for the heart primarily by a riveting Shropshire lad named William Withering, whose book *An Account of the Foxglove*, first published for five shillings a copy and featuring a painting of the purple foxglove as frontispiece, is still in print two centuries later.

Talented bagpiper and golfer was William Withering, avid botanist, bitter enemy of slavery and liquor, amateur Shakespearean actor, close friend to Erasmus Darwin and Ben

Franklin, interested in and respectful of folk remedy: it was during his travels through rural England visiting his patients that he heard of an old Shropshire woman who knew an herbal cure for faltering hearts, and he set himself to test the effects of foxglove distillate on more than a hundred patients, including himself.

"I prefer the leaves," he wrote in 1785. "These should be gathered after the flowering stem has shot up, and about the time that the blossoms are coming forth. The leaf-stalk and mid-rib of the leaves should be rejected, and the remaining part should be dried, either in the sunshine, or on a tin pan or pewter dish before a fire. If well dried, they readily rub down to a beautiful green powder. I give to adults from one to three grains of this powder twice a day ... it has a power over the motion of the heart, to a degree yet unobserved in any other medicine, and this power may be converted to salutary ends."

*

Because every part of *mearacan dearg* contains the glycosides digitoxin, gitoxin, and digoxin, distillates of foxglove were used as laxatives for centuries before Billy Withering realized its salutary ends; but because each of those glycosides is poisonous in large doses, many of the people given heroic doses of distillate of foxglove for their bowel troubles promptly died. The meticulous Withering listed the parade of symptoms in patients overdosed with foxglove powder: "vomiting, giddiness, confused vision, objects appearing green or yellow; increased secretion of urine, with frequent motions to part with it, and sometimes inability to retain it; slow pulse, even as slow as 35 in a minute, cold sweats, syncope, death." Which is why Withering prescribed tiny doses to his patients. Nearly a century later a German doctor named Traube arrived at an accurate measurement of effect: digitalis in doses smaller than two milligrams stimulates the heart muscle beneficially, but doses larger than two milligrams stimulates it too strenuously, to the point where paralysis often results.

In other words: a little poison is good for the heart.

*

My son Liam takes a little foxglove poison in the morning and a little at night. He takes a whole tablet of digoxin with his bowl of cereal and a half a tablet with his bowl of rice. It used to be that I would just put the pills on the table by his place in the morning but sometimes they would get swept to the floor by the flutter of the sports section, or they would wobble away crazily to hide under the fruit bowl, or they would be lost or mislaid or thrown in fury at taunting sister or brother, so my wife found a tiny wooden box for the pills, which protects them against loss or flinging, and also serves to remind her and me and Liam whether or not he has taken his pills, because when it comes to his medicine the kid has the memory power of a speck of dust, and he will airily claim to have taken them or not taken them based on, apparently, whichever possibility presents itself to his airy mind first, so if I am not sure he has taken the medicine I check inside the small green box. I have come to like the small green box very much, for complicated reasons, among them this: it holds a sliver of my son's salvation not once but twice a day.

I have taken, in recent years, to divesting myself of every Thing that I once thought meant so much to me, books and records and basketball jerseys and beach stones and love-letters and posters and paintings and knickknacks of every conceivable sort and shape and stripe, and I am lately down to a shoebox of photographs which to me are lovely shards of arrested time, but one Thing I will keep as long as I live, I hope, is Liam's little green box, the size and color of a hummingbird. It seems like an ark to me, a covenant, a tiny chapel, the two fitted pieces of it two hands met in prayer, two wings folded over a magic middle.

*

Let us consider other winged things. Birds have four-chambered hearts like ours but their hearts are bigger than ours, as a percentage of body weight, and faster than ours. The heart of a chicken beats four times faster than ours, the crow five times faster, the sparrow six times faster, the hummingbird nine times faster. A hummingbird's heart beats ten times a second. A hummingbird's heart is the size of a pencil eraser. A hummingbird is perhaps the most amazing thing there ever was. Consider the hummingbird closely for a long moment. *Joyas volardores,* flying jewels, the first white explorers in the Americas called them, and they had never seen such creatures, for hummingbirds came into the world only in the Americas, only here, nowhere else in the universe, more than three hundred species of them whirring and zooming and nectaring in a hummer time zone nine times removed from ours, their hearts hammering faster than we could clearly hear were our elephantine ears pressed to their infinitesimal chests.

*

Each one visits a thousand flowers a day. They can dive at sixty miles an hour. They can fly backwards. They can fly more than five hundred miles without pausing to rest. But when they rest they come close to death: on frigid nights, or when they are starving, they retreat into torpor, their metabolic rate slowing to a fifteenth of their normal sleep rate, their hearts sludging nearly to a halt, barely beating, and if they are not soon warmed, if they do not soon find that which is sweet, their hearts grow cold, and they cease to be.

Consider for a moment those hummingbirds who did not open their eyes again today, this very day, in the Americas: bearded helmetcrests and booted racket-tails, violet-tailed sylphs and violet-capped woodnymphs, crimson topazes and purple-crowned fairies, red-tailed comets and amethyst woodstars, rainbow-bearded thornbills and glittering-bellied emeralds, velvet-purple coronets and golden-bellied star-frontlets, fiery-tailed awlbills and Andean hillstars, spatuletails and pufflegs, each the most amazing thing you have never seen, each thunderous wild heart the size of a pebble, each mad heart silent, a brilliant music stilled.

*

The great American poet Pattiann Rogers, in a poem about hummingbirds, makes her lines swoop and slice, makes the poem *whirrrrrrrrrr* through the wild world just like the wee bird itself: *hovering in midair plummeting the light's most perfect desire the weaving twisting vision of red petal and nectar and soaring rump the rush of wing in its grand confusion of arcing and splitting spinning bloom of ruby sage breathless piece of scarlet sky ...*

*

Hummingbirds, like all flying birds but more so, have incredible enormous immense ferocious metabolisms. To drive those metabolisms they have race-car hearts that eat oxygen at an eye-popping rate. Their hearts are built of thinner leaner fibers than ours. Their arteries are stiffer and more taut. They have more mitochondria in their heart muscles. Anything to gulp more oxygen. Their hearts are stripped to the skin for the war against gravity and inertia, the mad search for food, the insane idea of flight. The price of their ambition is a life closer to death; they suffer heart attacks and aneurysms and ruptures more than any other living creature. It's expensive to fly. You burn out. You fry the machine. You melt the engine. Every creature on earth has approximately two billion heartbeats to spend in a lifetime. You can spend them slowly, like a tortoise, and live to be two hundred years old, or you can spend them fast, like a hummingbird, and live to be two years old.

*

The biggest heart in the world is inside the blue whale. It weighs more than seven tons. It's as big as a room. It *is* a room, with four chambers. A child could walk around in it, head high, bending only to step through the valves. The valves are as big as the swinging doors in a saloon. This house of a heart drives a creature a hundred feet long. When this creature is born it is twenty feet long and weighs four tons. It is waaaaay bigger than your car. It drinks a hundred gallons of milk from its mama every day and gains two hundred pounds a day and when it is seven or eight years old it endures an unimaginable puberty and then it essentially disappears from human ken, for next to nothing is known of the mating habits, travel patterns, diet, social life, language, social structure, diseases, spirituality, wars, stories, despairs, and arts of the blue whale. There are perhaps ten thousand blue whales in the world, living in every ocean on earth, and of the largest mammal who ever lived we know nearly nothing. But we know this: the animals with the largest heart in the world generally travel in pairs, and their penetrating moaning cries, their piercing yearning tongue, can be heard underwater for miles and miles.

*

Mammals and birds have hearts with four chambers. Reptiles and turtles have hearts with three chambers. Fish have hearts with two chambers. Insects and mollusks have hearts with one chamber. Worms have hearts with one chamber, although they may have as many as eleven one-chambered hearts. Insects have hearts that pump their version of blood, hemolymph, over and through all the organs in their remarkable bodies. Our hearts feed blood; their hearts bathe blood. Unicellular bacteria have no hearts at all; but even they have fluid eternally in motion, washing from one side of the cell to the other, swirling and whirling. No living being is without interior liquid motion. We all churn inside.

*

So much held in heart in a life. So much held in heart in a day, an hour, a moment. We are utterly open with no one, in the end—not mother and father, not wife or husband, not lover, not child, not friend. We open windows to each but we live alone in the house of the heart. Perhaps we must. Perhaps we could not bear to be so naked, for fear of a constantly harrowed heart. When young we think there will come one person who will savor and sustain us always; when we are older we know this is the dream of a child, that all hearts finally are bruised and scarred, scored and torn, repaired by time and will, patched by force of character, yet fragile and rickety forevermore, no matter how ferocious the defense and how many bricks you bring to the wall. You can brick up your heart as stout and tight and hard and cold and impregnable as you possibly can and down it comes in an instant, felled by a woman's second glance, a child's apple breath, the shatter of glass in the road, the words *I have something to tell you*, a cat with a broken spine dragging itself into the forest to die, the brush of your mother's papery ancient hand in the thicket of your hair, the memory of your father's voice early in the morning echoing from the kitchen where he is making pancakes for his children.

*

In the innermost recess of my old heart is a girl I call Emma, who was never born and never revealed her gender and never received her name except in my heart. *Imo pectore.* She was conceived ten years ago, a child of me and my wife and the mystery that flicks lives into being, and she lived for eight weeks inside my wife.

The child's heart beat: but she was growing in the wrong place inside her extraordinary mother, south of safe, and when she was eight weeks old she and her mother were rushed to the hospital, where her mother was operated upon by a brisk cheerful diminutive surgeon who told me after the surgery that my wife had been perhaps an hour from death from the pressure of a child growing outside the womb, that both mother and child would have soon died, the mother from the child growing and the child from growing awry; and so my wife did not die, but our mysterious child did.

Not uncommon, an ectopic pregnancy, said the surgeon. Serious but operable, no permanent damage to the mother.

Sometimes, continued the surgeon, sometimes people who lose children before they are born continue to imagine the child who has died, and talk about her or him, it's such an utterly human thing to do, it helps deal with the pain, it's healthy within reason, and yes, people say to their other children that they actually do, in a sense, have a sister or brother, or did have a sister or brother, and she or he is elsewhere, has gone ahead, whatever the language of your belief or faith tradition. You could do that. People do that, yes. I have patients who do that, yes.

And we did that, my wife and I, first with our daughter, who was two years old when we lost the ectopic child, and then with our subsequent sons, and sometimes now, years later, one of the three living children will say to me, about his or her sort of sister, *I wonder who she might have been*, but I find myself thinking *I wonder who she is*.

One summer morning, as I wandered by a river, I remembered an Irish word I learned long ago, and now whenever I think of the daughter I have to wait to meet, I find that word in my mouth: *dunnog,* little dark one, the shyest and quietest and tiniest of sparrows, the one you never see but sometimes you sense, a flash in the corner of your eye, a sweet sharp note already fading by the time it catches your ear.

7. *Gad*

God is not a person. God is not an idea. God is the engine. God is the beat. We are distracted by the word God. It gets in the way of the beat. Forget the word. It's only a word. It has a past; it comes from the ancient Hebrew word *gad,* which means to crowd upon or attack or invade or overcome. So the word we use today for the throb under and in and through all things is a verb. Sometimes we do things right. The ancient Jews got it right: they referred to God as *HaShem,* The Name. So many names through the centuries of human beings trying to sing along with the beat: *gott, khoda, khooda, gheu, emu, div, thes, deva, dyaus, deus, theos, dia, el, ilu, ilah,* so many words meaning the same thing: the center, the throb, the Heart. Forget the name of the Heart. Forget any and all images of the Heart, perceptions, conceptions, traditions, instructions. Cease to try to understand. Just listen. Just feel it humming hammering holy.

*

And we are distracted by the person of God: the young intense dusty confusing testy paradoxical devout prickly paranoiac thin tired relentless Christ.

Whatever else he was he was a human being with a human heart, atria and septae, mitral and ventral valves, sixty beats a second perhaps, or maybe forty beats a second, he was a calm man quite sure of his work, he was about his Father's business, or maybe ninety beats a second, he was terrified of what was to be, he lost his temper in the temple, he wept with fear in the garden at night, knowing he would be pierced and lanced, knowing he would be speared in the heart as he hung struggling to breathe, sour wine on his lips, the afternoon brooding and lowering over Golgotha, the Place of Skulls.

He too was once a fertilized egg doubling and redoubling itself, forming endocardial heart tubes, myocardium and epicardium, the cells of what would be his heart miraculously migrating and fusing and dividing into the genius engineering of the four magic chambers, his amazing new heart beating beneath his amazing mother's amazing heart after eight weeks, his mother the extraordinary teenage girl who said yes yes yes, as all mothers do, all their lives; and then mere moments later he is crying *Eloi! Eloi!* as he dies, he breathes his last, he yields up his spirit, his heart sludges to a halt on a cross on a bitter bleak afternoon; and then, three days later, in the oceanic black silence of the tomb in the garden, the tomb where no one had yet been laid, the tomb with the seal on the stone, the tomb redolent with myrrh and aloe and linen and spice, suddenly

There's a heartbeat,

And another,

And another,

And another ...

*

One of the most interesting men I ever met in this life is a tall craggy-faced cheerful man who travels the world collecting stories and talking to people. He is many things: husband, father, naturalist, writer, Zen priest. He has written books about cranes and sharks and fishermen and leopards and sandpipers and tigers and plovers and missionaries and thieves. Much else. A while ago we sat and talked for a long time about prayer and music and attentiveness and the shape and song of the heart. We talked about Zen meditation and Catholic mysticism and the wild holy songs of William Blake and the Hindu chants known as the *Rigveda*, the verses of wisdom and praise. In Hindu lore these chants have come down to us from the beginning of time, and are the cosmic reverberations of divine harmony; she or he who hears or speaks them hears or speaks, however tenuously or briefly, the music of God. Even the syllables of the *Rigveda* are holy and powerful, and the most potent of them all is *om*. As my friend remarked, when you chant and chant and chant *om*, again and again and again, your lips opening the *o* and kissing closed the *m*, to the point where you lose track of the time and the slight discomfort of your body in the chair and your pending and pressing duties and responsibilities and what time the grocery store closes and the sick child and the distant lover and the threatening weather and the silly song and the suffering road, and your mind drifts not up and away but *in*, into this one second, this one instant, a stunning *miracle* this one instant, an unbelievable gift, and you surf the single amazing miraculous unrepeatable inimitable instant like a boat on a surging sea, and you forget that you are chanting *om* again and again and again, you forget your usual and eternal and ethereal and exhausting consciousness of yourself, then you may find, said my friend, that when you surface again to sensibility, you have been chanting at exactly the pace of the beat of your heart.

*

How long has the human heart been the seat of the soul? Longer than human history is recorded. The fist of electric elastic ebullient endless energy in your chest was the distilled essence of character and spirit for the Sumerians, the Egyptians, the Greeks, the Thracians, the Romans, the Mayans, the Aztec, the Australians, the Celts. Four thousand years ago when a man or woman or child in Egypt died, his or her *ba*, the soul, traveled through the underworld through fire and cobras, to the halls of the jackal god Anubis, who weighed your heart against *maat*, the feather of Things As They Should Be. If your heart was too heavy or too light, it was eaten by monsters and you were doomed to sleep until the end of time. If your heart was evenly balanced, you were sent on into the light, where you could again enjoy the love of the living.

*

Consider why, all through history and in every sort of literature, the heart should be considered the seat of the soul, and not the head. What races when you are stimulated by love or fear? Not the head. In fact the governor upstairs generally freezes when faced by conundrum or coquette. The heart responds instanter. Which is why many American Indian cultures ate the hearts of their bravest enemies.

*

I watched a heart operation today. The patient and the surgeon and the assistant surgeon and three nurses were in the operating room and I was in an adjacent room watching a video feed. With me were surgeons from all over the world, here by invitation of a health care company.

The doctor on my right side is from France. We shake hands. He doesn't have much English and I have no French. I show him my notepad and pen and he smiles and says *ah, le journaliste.* The doctor to my left is from Australia. He speaks Australian, a smiling sunny language which takes me a minute to get the pace and rhythm of, but then we get along swell, and he is my cheerful technical guide through the subsequent operation, whispering entertaining comments here and there.

I compliment his absolutely lovely shimmering suit.

"Ya loike it, eh?" he says. "Oi love it but Oi never get to wear it at work. Oi wear it when Oi travel. Oi look better outside my country than Oi do innit."

Patient, age 33, has mitral valve failure. The surgeon opens the man's chest at 8:06 a.m. and his assistants pour cold water on the heart to cool it to 28 degrees centigrade. Assistant pours ice onto heart. Temperature drops to 10 centigrade. Surgeon waits for "myocardial tissue to stop wriggling."

Surgeon asks for size six thread. Nurse only has sizes four and five on hand.

Then the assistant moves a retractor the wrong way.

"This retractor is bothering the hell out of me!" says the surgeon. "You may have already injured the tissue!"

Surgeon cuts a triangle from the valve, stitches for a while, considers. He takes a stitch in the northeast corner of the valve. Worse. Surgeon sighs.

"On kids," he says casually, making conversation, "we use size seven thread."

Surgeon starts asking for length of operation every few minutes. He wants to be sure he doesn't have the patient open more than an hour without blood to his heart. The heart needs oxygen. Surgeon stitches southeast side. Considers. Stitches. Pauses. Moves tissue around. "Damn. Suture definitely distorted valve. Damn!" Takes out knot on northeast corner of valve. Takes out knot on southeast corner of valve. The ice has melted.

"Let's regroup," says the surgeon, and the assistant floods blood back into the heart. They wait a while. Then the blood is sucked out again and the surgeon goes back in. He ties new knots south and west. Time: 9:21 a.m. Stitching fast now, he closes heart up deftly, checks it for leaks, stitches last hole and ties off. 9:38 a.m.

Assistant pumps all air out of heart. Heart warms up again. Shudders into beat. Stops twice, shocked into starting again.

"He'll be happy with this heart," says the surgeon. "That's a good-looking heart."

"Good job," says assistant.

"You are either competent or incompetent. I am competent," says the surgeon. He steps away and the assistant closes up the patient. Time: 10:08.

Surgeon pops into adjacent room where I have watched the operation and we talk for a minute. He's wearing sneakers, I notice. He pours coffee and talks technique and history of operations. He tells me he has a second operation scheduled for noon.

After he leaves I sit and think what was most interesting about these 122 minutes of heart surgery, and I conclude that it is the sheer creativity of the operation—the volatile nature of it, the sense that there were successes and failures during it, the waxing and waning and waxing of the surgeon's elation, the feeling that he was in many ways making it up as he went along. Certainly there was vast technical skill at work—his stitching alone was amazing—yet really the operation was a creative act. He was painting, sculpting, writing, dancing, singing. He was, in a real sense, winging it. He invented the process as he went along. He applied vast experience and craft and desire and technique and intellect and grace and rudeness to a problem and solved it. But there was more to the operation than the solution to a problem. The surgeon built a new heart from the old one. He made a new thing in the world.

I talk about this to the Australian surgeon.

"Yeh, ya got the sense of it right," he says. "Now, any good surgeon could make a new heart out of an old one, sort of, but the interesting thing is this: no two surgeons would do it exactly the same way. Ya couldn't, you see. The patient's always different and every operation's sloightly different as well. The ingredients moight be the same but the cake's different every time out. Now *that's* interesting, isn't it?"

I agree that that's very interesting indeed.

We talk about the American surgeon who did the operation. The American surgeon is famous all over the world. He is said to be among the finest cardiac surgeons in America. He has founded and established and assisted and supported and visited and counseled and advised and procured money for heart clinics all over the world. In many ways he is a man of enormous influence, a man who has personally saved the lives of thousands of children, a man who has brought his talents to bear with stunning focus and effect, a man whose beneficial effect on the future of pediatric cardiology will be felt for a century.

I ask the Australian surgeon his opinion of the American surgeon.

"Well, he's a horse's ass," he says cheerfully. "And he has the personality of a desk. He's woidely disliked. But God gave him those hands. You can dislike a man but you must be honest about his gifts, and God gave that man those hands."

*

Here's a story. In 1945 two men were in the desert in Egypt digging for fertilizer. One man was named Muhammed and the other was Khalifah. They uncovered a red clay jar. At first the men decided not to break the jar for fear there were dark spirits inside, but then they considered that there might be gold inside, so in the eternal way of men considering that there might be some cash to be had from violence, Muhammed smashed the jar with his shovel.

Inside the jar were thirteen books made of papyrus. Muhammed wrapped the books in his cloak and took them home to his village, al-Qasr. At first Muhammed left the books in a pile of straw by the oven, from which pile his mother, in the eternal way of women considering that there might be some utilitarian use to be had from mannish muck, used some of the pages for kindling the fire and gave some others of the pages away to neighbors, among them a one-eyed outlaw named Bahij Ali.

After a while Muhammed gave the rest of the books he had left to a local priest named Basiliyus Abd al-Masih, who showed them to his brother-in-law, a teacher named Raghib Andrawus, who thought they might be valuable, and he then, in the eternal way of men interested in big cash, went to the city, taking them to Cairo, where he showed the books to a doctor named George Sobhi, who thought they might be valuable, and George Sobhi showed them to the government, which concluded that they were valuable, and in the eternal way of greedy governments everywhere, seized the books, and put them in the national museum, and eventually the government obtained all the rest of the unburned pages and books that had traveled from neighbors to dealers to collectors all over the world, all the pages except those toasted forever by Muhammed's mama, and now the pages are in the national museum in Cairo. All the pages are from the fourth century, and the stories they contain were originally written in Greek, and they tell of a mysterious man at the dawn of the first century, who said, among many other things in those books found by Muhammed and Khalifah one day in the desert:

The Kingdom is within you.
What is hidden from thee shall be revealed unto thee.

Love thy brother as thy soul.

Blessed is the man who has suffered; he has found life.

I am the light that is over them all.

I am the All; the All has come forth from me, and the All has attained unto me.

Cleave a piece of wood: I am there.

Raise up the stone, and ye shall find me there.

Seek, and ye shall find; he who seeks shall find, and he who knocks, to him it shall be opened.

The kingdom of the Father is spread out upon the earth, and men do not see it.

And many other things.

But this morning, as I ponder the light that is over all, and contemplate the vast universe of that which is hidden from me, and slowly cleave the wood of my own confusing confused heart, while grinning at Muhammed's mom, I remember one other haunting line from that pile of paper:

You that hath ears, let him hear this.

To which I say amen and then amen and then again amen.

8. Well, There Are a Lot of Stories

And there are all sorts of stories about hearts, and how hearts are brave or craven or both at once, and how hearts swell and leap, and shrivel and sigh and fail, and how people's hearts are in their mouths, and how we hold our hearts and other people's hearts in our hands, and how hearts break and are stunned and startled, and my heart is constantly being stunned and startled by the stories people tell me, so here are some of those stories. People will tell you the most amazing stories if only you ask.

*

One time I said to Dave tell me a story, and he told me about his patients in Alaska. Dave has patients from Barrow, which is the northernmost point in the United States and deep into the Arctic Circle, to Unalaska, which is in the Fox Islands deep in the Bering Sea near Russia, to Sitka, which is in the Alexander Archipelago, the wet soggy green southern tip of Alaska. He has patients in Akhiok and Elim and Huslia and Kipnuk and Kivalina and Kotzebue and Niuqsut and Nulato and Selawik and Shishmaref and Soldotna and Togiak and Tok and Toksook and Tununak and many many other alaskaplaces.

His patients are ages zero to fifteen. Some of his patients are less than zero. One time Dave flew to Bethel, on the Kuskokwim River near the Yukon Delta National Wildlife

Refuge, and a huge blizzard blew in and he was socked in for days without a change of clothing or a toothbrush. Not having a toothbrush really bothered him and so now when he travels he always carries a toothbrush in his pocket just in case.

Bethel has great salmon fishing and one grocery store and no sidewalks and about two thousand residents most of whom are Inuit or Upik or Athabascan and most of the rest of whom are public health service doctors and nurses working two-year stints to pay off medical school loans. When Dave landed that morning he got a cab from the airport to the town through the driving snow. The cabdriver was a Russian man who used to run a symphony orchestra in Vladivostok. When Dave got to town he discovered that dozens of dogsled racers and hundreds of their sled dogs were in town for the start of the Kuskokwin 300 sled dog race which runs fifty miles from Bethel to Akiachak and Akiak and Tuluksak and Bogus Creek and Kalskag and Pike Lake and back to Bethel, when it runs, which it wasn't running that day because of the blizzard. The sled dogs howled all day long. It was 10 degrees outside and children in shorts and shirts were playing soccer on the river. There being no way to see patients, on account of the blizzard, and not being a drinking man, Dave spent his Saturday night in Bethel with pretty much all of the other two thousand residents of the town and all the mushers in town for the race, watching Bethel High School's basketball team take on Barrow High's basketball team. Most of the spectators rode snowmobiles to the game. Most of the players on both teams were tattooed and most could dunk. Barrow's team, which had flown in to Bethel on a chartered flight, whupped on Bethel; it would go on to win the Alaskan state championship. The day after the game the Barrow team took a chartered flight home but a charter flight could not be found for a pediatric cardiologist, so Dave, furious that basketball outweighed babies' lives, had to stay in Bethel another night. That still makes me mad, he tells me. I could see a hockey team being more important than me, but a *basketball* team?

*

A priest tells me a story. He's a chaplain in a hospital. Two men are waiting for heart transplants at the same hospital. Both men are in and out of the hospital, their hearts deteriorating as they wait. Surgery and medicine can no longer help either man; they both need new hearts. Days go by, weeks, months, a year, two years. The men know each other and greet each other warmly and are friends in the country of the sick heart. Neither mentions their unspoken competition for the heart that may or may not arrive, still beating, from the recently vacated chest of its former owner. More time goes by. The men are in and out of the hospital. My friend the priest sees them every week. Finally one man's original heart fails and he dies. A few days later a heart arrives, on Good Friday, and it is transplanted into the second man's chest, on Holy Saturday, so on Easter Sunday he has new life.

Talk about resurrection, says my friend. Talk about resurrection.

*

A man who was a soldier tells me a story. He was a soldier a long time ago. He was far from home, on a beach in the Pacific where there had been a howling ferocious battle between two armies for more than a month. But, hell, he says, they weren't really armies at all. They were just bunches of boys, really. That's all. Boys with guns. All wars are fought by boys. There were about a hundred of their boys trying to hold the beach and about a hundred of our boys trying to take it.

We wanted that beach pretty bad. I disremember why. Well, they died and we died. Our guys fought like mad. We killed a lot of their guys and they killed a lot of our guys. There was no way off that island at that time and there was nobody coming to rescue us either. That's just the way it was for a while, there was no supply line and no reinforcements and no replacements and the guys just were under fire day and night for weeks. I think it was twenty-eight days they were under fire all the time. Well, there are a lot of stories from those days, most of which no one will ever know because the guys who could tell them are dead. There were a lot of guys died there. The other guys had mined the beach to begin with when they knew we were coming in and so even after we were there and bunkered in and fighting you would still lose guys just walking on the beach. I saw a lot of things on that beach that make you sick just to think about them. One time I found a heart on the beach, just sitting there in the sand, all raggedy and a mess. I didn't know if it was from a human being or not. It was just sitting there on the beach. I was in a hurry but I buried it. Didn't seem right to leave a heart there all naked on the beach. Kicked sand over it and ran. Haven't thought about that in fifty years, I bet. Not the kind of thing you want to think about. But there it is.

*

I think about the people I know with the absolutely largest hearts, people with a stunning capacity for endurance and grace and kindness against the most screaming terrors and pains. My mom and dad, for example, enduring the death of their first child at six months old, the boy the brother I never met dying quietly in his stroller on the porch in the moment that my mother stepped back inside to get a pair of gloves because the crisp brilliant April day was filled with a whistling cutting wind she comes back out to the porch pulling on her gloves and smiles to see Seamus asleep she chucks him under his fat chin and he stays asleep and she looks twice and her heart freezes.

Fifty years later after five more children and two miscarriages she is standing in the kitchen with her usual eternal endless cup of tea and I ask her: How do you get over the death of your child?

And she says, in her blunt honest direct terse kind way, You don't.

Her face harrowed like a hawk for a moment in the swirling steam of the tea.

*

Yes, I talk to Seamus, said my dad the other day. Not often. In times of stress or when I especially need his help. I've talked to him a lot lately. He listens. He intervenes with God. We only have one photograph of Seamus, you know. We didn't take as many pictures of our first-born as we should have. I guess we didn't think there was any hurry. In the picture we have he's pushing himself up on his arms and holding up his head, looking at us, wearing a little white cap. That's the picture I have in my head when I talk to him. The little kid in the white cap who left us a long time ago but keeps watching over us. Yes, I talk to him from time to time. Yes.

*

Or my college friend Danno who has the biggest heart I ever saw and who always makes me laugh except one night when I am washing the dishes he calls me from the hospital where his daughter is dying. She got hit by a truck and broke everything you can break and she just received the last rites. She just had a baby boy. Dan is holding his grandson in his arms at the hospital. The boy is two months old. I remember when this boy's mama was two months old. She slept in the top drawer of a rickety bureau. Her folks had about seven cents when she was born. All these years later they don't have much more than seven cents but they had three more children after Julie and Dan would say grinning *we are rich rich rich rich*, and he meant it, too, even though they were never a bit of rich, and his wife's been sick for years, and the black dog has chased through their family, and another child of theirs once had a fever so virulent and savage that it sent the boy into a wheelchair for a while, and Dan has worked so hard and so long and at so many jobs at once to support his family that his hair went bone white before he was thirty, and a piece of his back broke once and they didn't have enough money then to fix it so he wept himself to sleep every night for a year, but all through his ocean of pain he has grinned and laughed and sang, and never have I met a man with such a heart, and I love him dearly, and I tell him that on the phone, and he says I love you too you mangy mule, and I chant the names of all his old girlfriends to make him laugh, which he does, I can hear him laughing in the hallway of the hospital far away with his grandson sleeping in his arms, and then he says I hafta go, pray for Julie, and we hang up and I pray helplessly into the sink, into the bubbles and apple peels, I pray for him and his family to be rich rich rich rich and not rich rich rich, I pray down into the cups and forks, the crusts of pizza my children refuse to eat, which drives me nuts, but I say aloud to the soggy crusts *rich rich rich rich*, which makes me cry, and I wash off the crusts and dry them and carry them out to the grass for the crows to eat for some reason I don't understand that has everything to do with praying for Julie.

*

Or *here's* a braveheart story. A young thin grinning unbelievably black man who tells me that one day when he was eight years old he was minding his family's cows and goats and sheep when some older boys came running and said that men were shooting all the boys and men in the village. So we started running toward the forest, he says. When I got to the forest I tried to hide but the forest was full of people. I could not find my family. I waited in the forest all day for the shooting to stop but it didn't stop. When night came we heard the men on horses in the forest looking for us, so we went deeper into the forest. It seemed like the whole world was hiding in that forest. The night grew cold but we could not light a fire. In the morning we walked to the next village but the men raided that village too, and the people there ran into the forest, so the forest grew more crowded. We all kept walking, just to go. This went on for three days. In the villages every boy and man was killed, and every girl taken alive. Old men and old women were left alone. In the forest if you were lucky someone gave you something to eat, and if you were unlucky you ate from the trees. After five days the elders in my village sent word that all young boys and young men from our village who were in the forest must keep walking east toward the border. They knew that if we came back to the village we would be killed next time the soldiers came. So I did not see my family again for a long time. There were hundreds of us boys in the forest, ages six to nineteen. We walked all night and slept all day. Sometimes we killed a bird and ate it. I walked with my cousin and three boys from our village. We five walked together. You held the shirt of the boy in front of you and a boy held your shirt behind you. I lost my shoes and made socks from my sleeves. It rained a lot but the rain was warm. There were always hyenas. They were looking for weak people to eat. You would hear them laughing. You would hear lions also. They weren't so bad. You would find them sleeping in the road. If you slept in their territory that was bad for you. Sometimes when you were looking for a bush to sleep under you would find a lion or a leopard under that bush. It was a silent journey. Not many boys felt like talking. We knew we had lost our parents. It smelled like trees and flowers. I cannot remember every day. We walked for three weeks through the forest. I lost my cousin. Finally we came to the border between Sudan and Ethiopia, and that was the end of one journey, and the beginning of another, and after a long while I got to be here, and here I am talking to you.

*

Friends tell me stories of people whose hearts grew gray: of the woman in Mayo who took to the bed for three years, and the man in Donegal who took to the bed for a year, and the cousin of a friend who takes to the bed every winter when the rains begin, and I am reminded of Darby Ruadh of Aughinish, who took to his bed for a year for yearning love of a woman he saw in a river, and of Aoifê of Connacht, who took to her bed for a year, emerging only to change her stepchildren into swans, for which she was punished by being changed into a gray vulture, doomed to live on the wing as long as time endured; which is to say that she could never take to her bed until the end of the world, which is a long time to be deprived of a particularly Irish form of refuge, retreat, restoration, surrender, defiance, passivity, prayer, and sadness.

In Irish culture, taking to the bed with a gray heart is not considered especially odd. People did and do it for understandable reasons—ill health, or the black dog, or, most horrifyingly, to die during An Gorta Mor, the Great Hunger, when whole families took to their beds to slowly starve; and there are black days upon me every year when I cannot help but see those families in their skeletal beds, the wet wind snarling, the infant boy whimpering, the last moans of the mother, the father weeping silently, the daughter staggering up at the last to fold the arms of her family across their chests as bony as birds.

So many dead in the bed.

And in our time: I know a woman who took to her bed for a week after September eleventh, and people who have taken to their beds for days on end to recover from shattered love affairs, the death of a child, a physical injury that heals far faster than the psychic wound gaping under it. I've done it myself twice, once as a youth and once as a man, the first time in sheer confusion and the second time to think through a troubled time in my marriage. Something about the rectangularity of the bed, perhaps, or supinity, or silence, or timelessness; for when you are in bed but not asleep there is no time, as lovers and insomniacs know.

Yet, anxious, heartsick, we take to the bed, saddled by despair and dissonance and disease, riddled by muddledness and madness, rattled by malaise and misadventure, and in the ancient culture of my forebears this was not so unusual, it happened in every clan, a brother to the bed or a mother to the mattress for a day a week a month a year three years the rest of her allotted days; and ultimately what is there to wonder at in this? For from the bed we came and to it we shall return, and our nightly voyages there are nutritious and restorative, and we have taken to our beds for a thousand other reasons, loved and argued and eaten and seethed there, and sang and sobbed and suckled, and burned with fevers and visions and lust, and huddled and howled and curled and prayed. As children we all, every one of us, pretended the bed was a boat; so now, when we are so patently and persistently and daily at sea, why not seek a ship?

*

Or my friend Bernie who died a while ago. He was a grand man altogether. He was eighty years old. He was in love with his wife. They had eight children. He spoke fluent Gaelic and reverted to that ancient tongue when he got to telling stories late at night. He liked to sit by the fire with a blanket around his knees and tell stories. His parents had come from Ireland as teenagers. They didn't speak English until they got to America. His father worked in a copper mine. His mother was a maid. He was a star football player in college and then was about to be a star football player for a professional team when the war came and he went to the war. When he came home from the war he went to work building roads in the most remote places in the West and one time he went to a dance in the mountains and there was the most beautiful girl he ever saw surrounded by a pack of young strong guys and he made his way through the phalanx of young strong guys and danced with her and soon they were kissing and then they were married and then they had eight children. He worked the rest of his life building roads and telling stories and kissing that girl. When he died sixty years after he met that girl in the mountains she asked me to speak at his funeral. At the funeral I said a prayer in Gaelic, so that the language of his parents would wash over his body one last time, and then I held up my hands and talked about the way his huge strong bony gaunt gentle hands had cradled a football and hammered his brothers and tickled his sister and cupped his mother's face and clapped his father on the shoulder and wielded a shovel and pumped saws through firs and cedars and skimmed over the supple sweet skin of his wife and cupped his children and worked concrete and stone and wood and plaster and paint and were plunged in sand and sliced through the ocean and cleaned and washed and folded and dried and cooked and prayed and weren't his hands the story of the man? Weren't his hands always shaping the song of his heart?

*

Here's a braveheart story. A quiet man brown as a tree tells me he was in a war and his side lost so he had to leave his country and escape into the next country which he did even though he lost a foot in the war and had to hop across the border at dusk carrying his crutch. The country he escaped into was even worse off than his own country and people were being killed there if they wore eyeglasses or could read. You wouldn't believe the reasons people were killed there, he says. One time they killed all the doctors and nurses and teachers just because. Another time they killed everyone in a city because they decided cities were evil. They killed all the priests and nuns and monks too just because. So I concluded to escape that country also. I went through the forest and I got to the border and the soldiers caught me and they threw me in a prison. That prison was so far deep in the forest no one even knew where it was except the soldiers. It was all mud and blood there. Women and men were there and the men were all beaten and the women worse. I was blind then from the war and I was in a pit in the bottom of the prison. So I concluded to pray. I prayed for two weeks all the time except when the soldiers were hitting me. I did not expect a miracle to happen. No. That is not what praying is for. I was praying not to lose hope. I was praying to be calm and accept what would be. I was praying to be calm about what would happen. I did not know what would happen. After a while the soldiers let me go and I went to a refugee camp and then I went to another country and then I came to this country. That's a long story. In this country I learned how to fix things and found work fixing things and I met my wife and now we have two boys. They are intelligent boys. They listen to me sometimes when I tell them stories about the war and prison and the forest. I don't know what they think about those stories. I told them that I prayed in the pit in the prison. One time one son asked me if my prayers were answered. I said that prayers were not questions to be answered. It is a mysterious thing what prayers are. It is an interesting thing to me that everybody has prayers even if they don't have religions. That is a *very* interesting thing.

*

A friend writes: "I'm trying to live by heart, because it's the one human organ in which I've never lost faith. When brains break they usually seem to stay broken. When hearts break, though, a surprisingly frequent result is a torrent of newfound compassion. I'm so impressed by this that in my heart I don't feel angst or despair at all. I feel a need to stand by my heart's assessment, often against the endless evidence spewed at me by my head. Easy angst and despair feel dangerous to me— feel like assessments made by the head alone. To be born, in a headish manner of speaking, is to commence the long slow process of dying. But to be born is also to begin being alive in a body in a world—an incredible gift if, like me, you're incapable of giving birth to yourself or of creating a world. So why put it the head's way? My head tells me daily that I've been slowly dying for fifty years now and that I'll probably die painfully of cancer so it might not be a bad idea to slash my wrists while I've got the strength. But my heart tells me that it's immensely grateful for the whole unpredictable extravaganza that is life."

*

Here's a dark heart story. My neighbor's house burned to the ground last month with her in it. Her name was Vikki. She was fifty-four years old. She lived alone. She had two cats. She never married. Had no children. Was a bookkeeper but she was laid off and never got another job and never really came out of her house again.

We neighbors were discreet or cold or shy or ignorant or polite or distracted or respectful or whatever word fits the fact that we didn't know her and she didn't know us, which was, as one neighbor says, the way she wanted it.

Then came the fire. The flames rose twenty feet high and the long fingers of the brooding trees caught fire too and firemen sprinted and shouted and ambulances and fire engines and cop cars roared up and down the street and children wept and the adjacent houses were evacuated and the young woman in the house next to ours ran by me weeping with her two children cradled in her arms like footballs and a young policeman came to my door to warn us and I packed a box of photographs and passports and Important Papers and got ready to wake the children but then the young policeman came by again and said the fire was under control though the house was a total loss.

She died from the smoke, says the fire marshal. One cat burned also. The cat was in the living room. We think the other cat escaped. The fire started in the kitchen. We put a lot of water on the kitchen. That was the seed of the fire. Then it traveled into the attic and then it moved fast through the house. We put six thousand gallons of water on it. We had forty-two men there. Guys came from six towns around to help. We had men on it until dawn. The roof fell in finally.

Twenty years we were neighbors and I hardly knew her at all, says the neighbor next door. But that's how she wanted it. She'd do her shopping early in the morning so as not to talk

to people. I don't know what she was running from. She was
good at her job. She liked wind chimes and wind socks and
white wine and television and cats and dogs and cigarettes
and the daily newspaper. One time she had eight cats and two
dogs. She planted roses and hydrangeas but after she lost her
job she stopped tending to the flowers and her trees got all
ragged. She stopped eating and she got skinnier and skinnier.
She was just drinking water. I tried to bring her food but it
was no use. She said that nothing tasted good. She was some
kind of ill. She started opening her drapes later in the morning
and closing them earlier in the evening. She canceled the daily
paper and just got the Sunday paper and then came the fire.

Last night I stood by Vikki's fence. Her roses were in riotous
bloom. The ash was everywhere. Some of the ash was Vikki
and some was her cat. Some of the ash was Vikki's heart. After
the fire it rained for days. Ash washed into the river and down
to the sea. Sadness is a tide in every heart.

Her hawthorn trees are high and wild now. Once, long
ago, the people who lived on our hill used hawthorn ash to
make face paint for dances to drive away their sadness. They
would make a vast fire and whirl around it all night long and
in the morning when you washed the ashes from your face
you were clean and new and your sadness had died in the fire.

*

One last story: before the British novelist and poet Thomas
Hardy died, he left instructions that his heart be buried in
the church graveyard at Stinsford, in his beloved Dorset,
in keeping with an ancient tradition in English culture, in
which the heart returns to the place where it entered the
world. On Hardy's death, in 1928, the local veterinarian
removed Hardy's heart, put it in a biscuit box, left it on his
kitchen table, and repaired to the local pub for a pint of

bitter. When he returned he found the box empty and his cat looking almighty satisfied. He shot the cat and buried it in the churchyard under Hardy's gravestone.

Whenever I get all emotional and literary about hearts as metaphors, or speechlessly wowed by the actual technical muscular hematological genius architectural engineering of actual bloody electrical hearts, I think of Hardy's heart getting eaten by the cat, and this makes me grin, partly because I like stories where snotty cats get their oughts, but partly too because the story forces me to remember that hearts are just hearts, wet muscles relentlessly slamming blood into tubes. Most hearts work like mad for years and years, and then eventually they all fail, and when they are done working they are meat, and they get eaten, by cats or by worms or microbes or whatever.

But what *verbs* they were when they were working, what amazements, what miracles, what stories!

9. A Heartful of Patients

It's hard to actually meet Dave. He doesn't do email for fun and he's not much for notes and letters and cards and he only returns phone calls about or from his patients or the parents of his patients and he only makes appointments about or with his patients and the parents of his patients. So writing about Dave, which entails, ideally, spending some time with him, and talking to him, and asking questions, and listening to stories, and eliciting anecdotes, and checking facts, and poking after his ideas and convictions and epiphanies—well, that approach presents an interesting little moral dilemma, for every minute Dave spends with me, answering questions and telling stories, is a minute he is not with one of his patients, or his wife, and inasmuch as Linda has much the better claim on what free time Dave has, and inasmuch as many of his patients hover between life and death, it would be a remarkably selfish writer who would pester Dave for time for what is, ultimately, a project that does not directly save or heal a child with a heart problem.

You will say, as I have, to myself, does the man not have any free time? Does the man not savor the cinema and savor the wit and grace of his bride and climb mountains and run with the dogs and indulge in a bucket of beer here and there on a hot day and enjoy the theater and wade in a creek and catch a ball game and read a riveting novel and maybe once in a while for no reason whatsoever other than mammalian joy in being alive simply laze in the grass in the broad light of summer counting the sparrows who do not sow nor do they reap?

And I report to you that he does these things so seldom that essentially he does not do many or even most of the things that you might expect your average fifty-year-old healthy American man to do. I mean, yes, of course he eats and sleeps, and he *says* he makes out with Linda sometimes, although that is not something you can politely ask for confirmation or documentation on, and he *says* he reads sometimes, and he *says* he takes a vacation for a couple days around a cardiology conference once a year though both he and Linda have to stop and think for a minute about where it was they went last year (*o yeah, Colorado!*), but most of the time Dave is Doctor Dave, that's what he does, that's who he is, he is what he does, and he does it, or *is* it, pretty much seven days and nights a week, many of those nights on call, many of those nights the sort of nights, as Linda says, when her conversation with Dave is a terse *not going to make it home tonight* message in the phone, and many of those nights the sort of night where Dave prowls the halls of the hospital with a heartful of patients.

I wonder sometimes if Dave isn't a sort of priest, really, and Linda a sort of nun—their lives turned wholly to service, given over utterly to other people, their talents and time and character placed on the altar of the communal good. Such an admirable endeavor, too, the commitment and dedication of the priest or nun, the doctor or nurse or teacher or mother who gives *every* ounce of her or his energy and creativity and talent to saving health and hope among his or her broken human cousins.

But exhausting beyond articulation, no? Draining beyond measurement. Draining even beyond self-comprehension. How long could you pour yourself out before your self is dissolved? How much pain can you witness or carry?

I think about this all the time. I find myself staring at the shoulders of counselors and priests and doctors and mothers, to see what the weight looks like. I find myself thinking that most people sure are extraordinary. I find myself thinking, as I get older and less cocky and less sure and more merciful and more hip to the fact that everyone has scars on their hearts or will, and everyone carries loads or will, and everyone carries their load alone or will, that maybe all people are extraordinary, whether or not I see that clear, and that my seeing it or not seeing it has nothing to do with the reality of grace under duress, which is pretty much the story of the human race. Love carries a lot of pain in its chest.

*

Here's Dave's day. Ready? "Up at 4:45, don't need alarm clock. Shower, cup of chai tea, drive 22 miles from woods to city, get to hospital, check fax machine for EKGs of kids, check computer for vital signs of kids, EKGs and vital signs taken during the night of most of the kids under my care, then to the intensive care unit, check X-rays for kids going sour, then do rounds, sickest kids first and work your way down. Appointments begin at eight or nine in the morning, depending. Have another cup of tea. Some days we have committee meetings and all of us review cases together. There's usually a surgery. Sometimes two. There are a lot of phone calls and interruptions all day long. Some days I have appointments all day. Some days I am on the road for clinics. I get home at seven or eight at night, unless there's a reason for me to stay at the hospital. There's a reason to stay fairly often. Two or three nights a week, maybe. There's a room we can sleep in. If I'm not going to make it home I call Linda. She says she can tell by the tone of the phone ringing if I'm not going to make it home. If I do get home for dinner she's usually waiting for me. We eat together more than you might think. I try to read for an hour and we get to bed early, nine or ten maybe. Takes me about twenty seconds to get to sleep. I never have had much of a problem getting to sleep, I have to say. That's a blessing for a doctor. I'd make that a prerequisite for a medical career if I could."

*

Dave's office manager at the Children's Cardiac Center of Oregon is named Kathy. She is from Arkansas. At nineteen and a half years old she was married and a mother. At twenty and a half she was a mother again.

Her husband beat her again and again and again and again and again and again and again and again and again and again and again and again and again and again and again and again and again and again and finally she took her two small children and got on a bus in Little Rock, Arkansas, and rode three days and nights to Portland, Oregon, where she lived with her sister for a while and then she got a room in a house where the kitchen was upstairs in the landlady's room.

That was one tiiiiny kitchen, Kathy says, but we made do.

I got my children into school, she says, and then I ruminated as to what I would do.

I had ambitions, she says. I went to college and earned my bachelor's degree in psychology and then I went to the hospital school here to study to be a technician, which I did become, here at the hospital, for eventually nineteen and a half years. Then I announced my imminent retirement from that position, and at that time Dave asked me to consider working in his office.

Well, I went home and thought about that. I took a long trip back to Arkansas to see friends and family. I drove. I took myself some time.

Then I accepted that position in Dave's office. At the first I was to be in charge of all the machines, and there are many machines and computers and service contracts and maintenance and complex operations, but relatively soon thereafter Dave asked me to consider managing the office, and I accepted that position, and that is what I do now, I manage the operation, which is not part of the hospital, but a standalone entity housed here in the hospital.

Well, of course we have cordial professional relationships all over the hospital, and with other hospitals and clinics and all, but I make pains to state that we are ourselves. We work with all ages of patient from people in their fifties or so down to the infants. We have far more children than any other sort of patient. That's because of referrals and word of mouth and people talking to people about the work we do. We don't advertise or anything. That's not the way we do things. One family tells another sometimes. Or more often the doctors and nurses we work with send their patients to us.

We always have a lot of patients. Yes we do. All over the West, California all the way to Alaska. All over the world really. We have worked on thousands of hearts. Yes we have. Thousands. And I believe we will be working on many more hearts in the years to come. Thousands.

*

Dave's business manager at the Children's Cardiac Center of Oregon is named Michele. Michele started working with the Center eighteen years ago, quit coming to the office to raise her kids but kept doing the office billing from her home, and now that her kids are twenty and fifteen and thirteen and twelve she comes into the office again to do the work, although she is also now the founder and president of her own medical billing service company which employs fifteen people and serves forty-four doctors and demands that Michele have her cell phone on her person twenty-five hours a day, as she says. Michele is a brisk alert woman with a quick smile and quick eyes and a quick mind, and considering she knows more about how the Center works than anyone else, and has worked with Dave for thirteen years, one day I persuade her to leave her cell phone in the other room and talk to me about Dave, which she does.

Dave struck me right from the first as an extremely personable man, she says. He has always been really just down to earth. He gets very close to his patients. He gets closest to the ones who are doing the worst. And, you know, after thirteen years of children with the worst sorts of heart problems, a lot of patients have expired on Dave. Which is wearing. He's vulnerable. He has no walls. He connects more than any doctor I've ever seen and I have seen great doctors. He's more tired now than he was in the beginning, that's for sure. Which, considering he sees some eight hundred patients a year, you can see why. I mean, he's seen some seven thousand patients, I bet, and so many of those were little kids right on the edge. So I can see him retiring before the others. Dave always wants to learn, and he's very much an outdoors guy, and I could see him doing something utterly different than medicine. Building canoes or something. There's a lot of emotional wear and tear in this work. Not to mention the sheer number of hours. And he goes on the road too, in our clinics, he goes all over Oregon and Washington, to the hospitals that have no pediatric cardiologists. He pops a gasket sometimes when he's completely exhausted, but that's very rare. The way to tell that Dave is upset is when he gets quieter and quieter. The quieter he gets the worse it is.

*

In the two examining rooms that Dave uses at the Children's Cardiac Center of Oregon there are corkboards crammed and filled and overflowing with photographs of the children he has saved. The children and their parents send him photographs all the time. They also send him invitations to graduations, birthday parties, weddings, bar mitzvahs, bat mitzvahs, confirmations, first communions, baptisms, Christmas parties, picnics, barbecues, and gatherings of every other imaginable sort, but mostly he gets photographs. There are photographs of children playing guitars, basketball, baseball, soccer, and hockey. There are photographs of children hiking and fishing and howling with laughter at Disneyland and Sea World. There are children in front of Christmas trees and birthday cakes. There are school photographs. There are prom photographs. There are graduation photographs. There are photographs of children in playgrounds and school plays and bunny suits. There are children in Halloween costumes. There are children in pigtails and ponytails and bathing suits and first-day-of-school clothes. There are many photographs of children at the beach. There are many photographs of children in swimming pools. There are many photographs of beaming shirtless children pointing to their chests and on each chest being pointed to proudly there is a scar running from the base of the throat nearly to the belly button.

There are hundreds of photographs, so many that the ones with frames propped on the counters are all crowded together and the ones pinned and taped to the corkboards have long ago spilled over the edges of the corkboard onto the clean white walls.

*

Like all modern hospitals, Emanuel is today a vast technological city teeming with expertise and expense and electricity and energy, but like all hospitals its birth was poignant and personal: it was the brainchild of an evangelical minister named Carl Johan Renhard, pastor of the First Immanuel Church of Portland, who started it in 1909, in a narrow tall old house on Taylor Street in which the nurses lived on the third floor and surgeries were scheduled for the few hours every day when the Reverend Renhard, a strapping former Nebraska farm boy, was free to carry the patients up and down the stairs.

*

Linda McIrvin tells me a story. She and Dave were living in Maine. She was a nurse and Dave was beginning his practice as a pediatric cardiologist. One day he sees a family in his office. The patient is a boy named Sam Shorette, age ten, with Down's syndrome. He needs a mitral valve replacement. Dave explains this to the boy's parents, who reply that they will talk it over with their son and let Dave know what the son decides.

"For once, Dave was speechless," says Linda.

Sammy said yes and he had the surgery and it worked.

"One Sunday after that," Linda continues, "they invited us to their house for dinner. They lived in a farmhouse that was two centuries old and it was heated with a woodstove that was a century old. To find their house they said to look for the mailbox that said Shorette but every single mailbox up and down the road said Shorette. We found the house eventually. All the kids and grandkids from up and down their road came for dinner, and it seemed they were all related to Sammy somehow, and it was clear that they all loved that boy with all their hearts. His parents insisted we bring our dog in the house, and all during dinner our dog chased their cat around the furniture, under the table, in and out of the house, etc. The parents just laughed. It was a talkative, noisy, happy clan.

"They asked us to attend their church with them, in the city, so one Sunday we dressed up in our finery and arrived at their church, which turned out to be filled with retarded people like Sammy. It was the most entertaining church service either of us ever saw. The congregation felt very free to talk with the minister throughout the service. At one point the minister asked if anyone there knew where Sodom and Gomorrah was, and a man called out that yes, he knew: Sodom and Gomorrah were in Falmouth, Maine, just outside Portland. That still makes me laugh.

"After the service everyone came up to Dave and said with delight: *You're Sammy's doctah!*

"After we left Maine, we stayed in touch with letters and Christmas gifts and occasional phone calls. In April they called to tell us that Sammy died. His mom said she and her husband were alternating between tears and laughter. Later she wrote: 'I know you only knew him when he was little, but he did grow into a wonderful young man, loving and kind. Of course he had his moments ...'

"Included with the letter was a compact disk. It turned out that they'd met a country singer, way up in Maine, and he and Sammy got to be the best of friends. 'Sammy loved to sing every chance he could,' his mom wrote us. 'The Word says to make a joyful noise and he could do that with gusto ...' After Sammy died the country singer wrote a song called Sammy's Song and he recorded it and all the profits from that song go to the Special Olympics. So Sammy's still singing, sort of."

*

I wonder about doctors as players in moral theater: soldiers of a sort, battling death, the most consistent and insistent of enemies; wild lovers of a sort, throwing themselves headlong into relationships of terrific intensity that often end in disaster.

And this makes me think too that we are all of us players in small moral theaters all the time, theaters for the most part with an attendance of one or two, theaters playing stories that only those people will see or know. The moral life is conducted far more in mundane moments rather than momentous movements.

But of course no moment is mundane, and we make moral choices all day long, with only ourselves as witness.

*

Linda McIrvin tells me another Maine story, about a boy named Graham Morissette. She and Dave met him when he was nine months old. He had pulmonary stenosis. Dave arranged for a balloon dilation, which fixed the problem. After Dave and Linda moved to Oregon they stayed in touch with Graham and lots of cards and photographs and drawings went back and forth through the mails. As Graham grew up he decided he wanted to be a pediatric cardiologist like Dave. He was sure he remembered Dave from the procedure although he was less than a year old when it happened. At Halloween he went trick-or-treating as a pediatric cardiologist. When Graham was six years old he got leukemia. He fought it and it went into remission and then it roared back and he had a bone marrow transplant with marrow from his sister but the leukemia kept on coming and when Graham was about to die the Make-A-Wish foundation contacted the family and Graham asked for a hot tub so after he was gone the family could sit in it and watch the stars. He also asked his parents for a golden retriever puppy like the golden retrievers that Dave and Linda had. Four days before he died he got his golden retriever puppy. He named the puppy Finely because he finally got his puppy. He died on Christmas Eve, 1996. He was eight years old.

*

One day I meet Dave for an hour—a crack in his day opened in part by a series of fortunate coincidences (not on call, no patient in intensive care, no patient conference scheduled, no prospect of sudden patient airlifted down from Alaska) and in larger part by the shy engineering of Linda, who picks him up at the hospital in their truck, their dogs hanging out the windows, and brings him across the city to a picnic table where we talk until his cell phone rings and he has to go. But before he goes I ask him to tell me some stories about some patients and he talks like this:

The worst aortic valve I ever saw was in a boy two weeks old. He needed a valve replacement. He had surgeries at two months, two years, five years, and ten years. That was one tough kid. He didn't make it.

Or here's a story: Jeremy. He's twenty years old now. Had surgery when he was seventeen. All he wants to do is drive his snow machine. He needed a valve job in his heart. But the thing with him was that we knew for a number of reasons that he wouldn't get or take medication regularly, and we thought giving him a mechanical valve would just end up clogging up, so we gave him a tissue valve—we built a new valve out of the tissue he had. Well, I didn't. The surgeon did. He did a good job. Jeremy made it. He's probably out on his snow machine right now as we speak.

Or the kid from Trinidad we fixed, or the kid with Down's syndrome who had a hole in his heart, or the kid from Russia. There's a group called Healing the Children that started in about 1980 with a girl from Guatemala who needed a heart operation. Now they have fifteen chapters in more than twenty states and maybe fifty countries. We work with them through a partnership with a hospital. The hospital sets aside thousands of dollars a year for the program as a community service and we choose four or five kids a year. We could blow the whole budget on one kid who needs major work or we could do quick and dirty work on four or five kids. So we screen them carefully. We want to make the most use of our resources. Something we can do quickly, just in and out.

The kid from Russia was one of those. His mom was a dentist making about six dollars a month. The family lived in a tenement downwind from a nuclear testing site. Six kids *on their floor in the apartment building* had heart lesions. Makes you wonder. The kid needed a tetralogy repair. He came to us when he was three years old, very blue and thin, and after we fixed him it seemed like he gained about ten pounds a day. That was four years ago. He's doing fine, I guess. If we never see kids again that's good.

*

Tell me about more patients, I say. Free-associate. Just wing it.

I had identical twins once, he says. They made it. They're five years old now, I think. They don't live too far from here. They live out toward the woods.

Tell me about a girl. First one who pops into your mind.

Tessa, says Dave. She had a single ventricle. Her parents were bikers. They raised horses down in southern Oregon. Her mother had a plastic leg and her dad, Ivan, who was the nicest man you ever met, he was about six foot twelve. Enormous man. Played football for the University of Southern California. Nicest guy. She made it.

Tell me about a boy. How about kid who made it through college?

Hmm, Brandon, he says. Business major. Fraternity guy at the University of Oregon. Mature beyond his years, that kid. Sometimes I think that going through all this stuff when you're a kid really gives you perspective. Kids with congenital heart disease are much more mature than other kids.

Tell me a kid you have right now. A little kid.

Kelby. Four years old. Pulled his catheter two days ago. He calls me Doctor McGoo.

Tell me a kid you had from abroad.

I had a kid from China once, says Dave, and he'd had a valve job when he was an infant, but no one knew what *kind* of valve job, there were no records of the operation or anything. *That* was a memorable case. He made it.

Tell me a bizarre story.

I have a young woman named Amelia, says Dave, who had a heart and lung transplant, and in the bed next to her in the hospital I found a friend of mine from high school. His heart gave out on him and he had to have a transplant. Great guy. I hadn't seen him for years and years. That was unusual. He made it. She did too. She's in college now here in Portland.

How about a kid from the wrong side of the tracks?

I had a kid named Dave, says Dave. He was a gang member. He needed aortic repair. He made it. Quit the gang too. He's twenty now. His dad's name was Noel Christmas and his sister's name was, no kidding, Mary. Can you believe it? Mary Christmas, daughter of Noel. You wonder how Dave got such a goofy name as Dave. My mom says she named me after Davy Crockett, but I don't know. She might be teasing me there.

*

It's a lovely afternoon, hot but breezy, the perfect Oregon summer late afternoon, the very reason people live in Oregon, and I keep asking Dave questions.

How much longer are you going to do this? I ask.

Not much longer, he says, in that brisk direct straight honest friendly crisp quick way of his. A year or two, I'm thinking. You burn out. It isn't the physical exhaustion. The physical exhaustion doesn't bug me. You can recover from that pretty quick. It's the children. It adds up. I mean, there's a kid I have now, Grant, he's seven years old and he's had eight surgeries. He's the toughest kid in the world, and his parents are the nicest folks in the world, but still, eight surgeries in seven years ... or there's Declan, in Alaska, he's six years old now, he's probably not going to make it unless he gets a transplant. I've had a lot of Declans. There are so many Declans. You remember the ones who die. You don't remember the ones who make it. Well, you remember some of the ones who make it. I tend to remember the ones who are ferocious fighters. I don't know why.

I'm at the point where as soon as the parents come in with their infant I look at the kid's face and I can mostly tell if he's going to make it or not. I get tired of knowing as soon as I see a kid for the first time that he's not going to make it, or that it's going to be a long road to maybe. I get tired of being the guy who in the next thirty minutes has to smash the life these people expected and hoped for. That wears on you after a while. It's that look in the parents' faces when you tell them their kid won't be normal. It's getting to be a bigger pill than I can swallow.

You would think that the longer you do this kind of work the more tricks you find, the more ways to bypass the worries, but it doesn't work that way.

What will you do after you quit doing pediatric cardiology? I ask.

I've thought about that, he says, smiling. Work in a free clinic maybe. Build a boat or a log cabin, something in the woods. We'd probably move to Colorado and live in a small town in the mountains. Linda wants me to get into politics, to be a city councilman or something. Which would be fun. But you know what I've always wanted to do? It sounds crazy, but I'd love to be a part-time junior high science teacher. *That* would be cool. All kinds of science. Biology mostly. Special focus on the heart.

Are you happy with the career you chose? I ask.

O yes, he says, without the slightest hesitation. Yeah. I helped some kids out.

10. How We Wrestle Is Who We Are

When my son was little, and all this was happening to him, all this editing and twisting and icing and stitching and worrying and weeping and beeping and not sleeping, I used to lie awake thinking about what I would tell him about this time. Someday, if he lived, he would ask me what happened then, and I would have to answer him with all the honesty and eloquence demanded of love.

This finally happened a month ago. We had a moment alone, which is rare, and we were sitting at the dining-room table having a burping contest and he suddenly said:

Explain to me my heart stuff?

Well, essentially you were born with three chambers in your heart and you need four.

What's a chamber?

Like a room for pumping blood. They're little but if you don't have four you lose.

Where did the other room go?

I don't know. Good question.

So Dave fixed me?

Dave and some other people.

How did they do that?

They opened your chest and moved things around so your heart worked better. They couldn't add a fourth chamber so they tinkered with veins and things and built you a new engine. Essentially.

Did they take my heart out?

No. They hooked it up to a machine and the machine kept it going during the operation, while they worked on things around the heart. Essentially.

How long was I plugged into the machine?

Ninety minutes, twice.

Which is how long?

Figure it out.

Pause.

A hundred and eighty minutes.

Yup.

Which is three hours.

Yup.

So am I three hours behind everyone else?

Pause.

Dad. Am I in a different time zone?

Yup.

Cool.

Yup.

*

A few days ago he and I were sitting at the picnic table out front in the roaring light of a summer morning here, and I asked him what hearts do.

Well, dad, he said, they pump your blood. They help you run. They slow down when you are sleeping. They make a really deep sound like the bass guitar in a band. When I am like thirty or forty years old I'll get another heart, maybe with a San Antonio Spurs logo on it. I don't think about my heart unless I'm sitting down. Sometimes I think about my heart when I am in bed trying to fall asleep. To be honest I think my heart is pretty much the same as other guys' hearts. It's not all that different. I have a certain kind of heart, that's all. If I don't get into professional basketball I might be a heart doctor like Dave. Or maybe I'll be an artist. I could do all three. I could play ball during the winter and then be a doctor and artist in the summers.

You could do that, I say.

Yeah, that'd be cool, he says.

*

One time when he was about five years old he shuffled down to breakfast, his stuffed pig under his arm like a football, and we got to talking about our dreams, and he noted that he often dreamed of heaven, which he figured made sense because he had been in heaven before he was born.

You remember heaven? I ask.

O yah, I remember that heaven, he says. God is there all the time. He is a really big guy. He is naked. He has a black beard. He is laughing all the time. He's a funny guy. He has really big hands. He's a really big guy. He's bigger than you, dad. I was not scared. No. Because he was laughing all the time. Yah, I remember that. O yah.

*

I remember packing his bag for the hospital. First surgery. If all goes well he'll be there about a week, says Dave. I pack for a week: One pair cotton pajamas with flap. One pair cotton socks. One blanket, cotton. One blanket, wool. One bag of diapers. One bag of wipes. One Junior Policeman badge from local police force. One Zuni bear fetish with two magic pebbles. He is sleeping as I am packing. He is snoring like a walrus. My wife carries him out to the car in the pelting rain. I carry his bag. The bag is black and the sky is black and the street is black and my heart is black.

*

I remember thinking that the operations would either work or not work and he would either live or die. There was a certain clarity there. I used to crawl into that clarity at night. I spent a lot of time thinking about him dead, about his small coffin, about what I would miss, about the extra bed, about his clothes, about his favorite stuff. Would I put his stuffed pig in his coffin with him or keep it so I could hold it sometimes?

I used to think what if they don't fix him all the way and he's a cripple all his life, a pale thin kid in a wheelchair who has crises?

What if his brain gets bent during all this and he ends up bad retarded?

What if he ends up alive but without his mind at all?

What if his brain and his body never grow up at all?

What then?

Who would he be?

Who would I be?

Would he always be what he might have been?

Would I love him still?

It's easy to love someone healthy and happy. What if I couldn't love him?

What if he was so damaged that I prayed for him to die?

Would those prayers be good or evil?

I don't have anything sweet or wise to say about those thoughts. I can't report that I found new courage in God, or that God gave me strength to face my fears, or that my wife's love saved me, or anything cool and poetic like that. I just tell you that I had those thoughts, late at night, in the dark, and they haunt me still. I can't even push them across the page here and have them sit between you and me unattached to either of us, for they are bound to me always, like the dark fibers of my heart. For our hearts are not pure; our hearts are filled with need and greed as much as with love and grace; and we wrestle with our hearts all the time. The wrestling is who we are. How we wrestle is who we are. It never stops. We are never complete. We are verbs. What we want to be is never what we are. Not yet. Maybe that's why we have these relentless engines in our chests, driving us forward toward what we might be.

*

We love so helplessly. We can't control our love or understand it or even articulate it much beyond the banal. And there are so many forms and levels and shapes and flavors and speeds and depths and topographies and landscapes and colors and musics of love that the default cultural concept of love as romance only is a willful cultural addiction to microcosm. Romance is a small sea in a vast ocean. The heart leaps in so many directions at once.

*

What might we be, as a species, in the years to come? O what, O God tell me, o people tell me, o friends and lovers tell me, o enemies tell me, o come clear to me in the entrails of birds and the fleeting tails of stars, what we might be if we rise and evolve, if we reach and leap, if we deepen and sing, if we come further down from the brooding trees and out onto the smiling plain, if we unclench the fist and drop the dagger, if we emerge blinking from the fort and the stockade and the prison, if we smash the bricks from around our hearts, if we cease to stagger and swagger, if we peel the steel from our eyes, if we yearn and learn, if we do what we say we will do, if we act as if our words really matter, if our words become muscled mercy, if we grow a fifth chamber in our hearts and a seventh

and a ninth, and become as if new creatures arisen from our
shucked skins, creatures become what we are so patently and
brilliantly and utterly and wholly and holy capable of ...

*

What then?

*

It's a glorious crisp sunny afternoon in Oregon, and I just
saw an osprey go by like a flying boat, and the cedar trees
are whistling waaay above me, and the first swifts are out,
jousting with the last swallows, and I am sprawled in the
grass thinking about Dave, and hearts, and what human
beings might be if we ever actually rise to our own sweet wild
possibilities, and I conclude that I am concluded, that I have
nothing more to say of import at the moment about hearts
and Dave and human beings, so I sprawl here in the grass
pondering what sort of ritual sacramental ceremony might
be apt now, at the end of a labor of love like this skinny book
has been, and Liam wanders out onto the grass and sprawls
companionably with his dad, and he and I decide to amble
and peramble, he and I, dad and boy, boy and dad, uphill to
the wine shop, and when we have achieved the peak of the
hill whereupon God has placed the wine shop, we shall enter
therein, Liam and me, me and Liam, me telling Liam not
to make any sudden movements in the wine shop or touch
anything or else there will be hubbub and breakage and daddy
taking out a seventh mortgage, and then we will purchase
us the best bottle of pinot noir in the store, and thereafter
shamble and shuffle home, and once home we shall lie on
the lawn and have a glass of the best, that is *I* will, not Liam,
although he can dip his finger in and have a taste if he wants
to and make that wizened scrunched wriggly face he makes

when he has a fingertip of wine, which I let him do when he wants, even though he is only ten years old, because life is short, and wine maketh merry the heart, and miracles happen all the time, miracles like his existence, and his face as round as a basketball, and his renovated heart, so for this holy boy, and for great generous gentle doctors like Dave, and all other miracles understandable and inexplicable, like wives and daughters and osprey and wine, I say amen and then amen and then again amen.

Thanks & Sources

Laaawd, the number of people to thank—you would think that no one could ever write even a thin intense odd little book without the help of about a thousand people.

You would be right.

So my heartfelt thanks to Dave McIrvin, who saved my son, and Albert Starr, who saved my son, and Hagop Hovaguimian, who helped save my son, and Dave Farris, who helped save my son, and Mary Jo Rice, who helped save my son, and Richard Lowensohn, who hauled my sons wet and wriggling into the wild world, and Liam Doyle, who *is* my son, who is a really cool kid.

And Joey Doyle and Lily Doyle, who are also really cool kids. And their mother my dear friend Mary Miller Doyle, who made our children in the holy cave of her belly, and brought more strength and grace and courage and love to bear on fear and confusion and travail than I ever thought humanly possible. Most remarkable woman I ever met, and I don't understand her one bit at all. And my niece Mary Eulalia Miller, who is now a doctor and was a huge help to me on technical medical matters in which I was a total mule, and Linda McIrvin, who is the patron saint of this book and helped me open doors and told me many stories and who has the coolest smile you ever saw, and Lil Copan, who poked me to do this book and now I owe her a bottle of the best red wine, and Kathy Reed, who is Dave's office manager and a brave cool woman, and Michele Anderson, who is Dave's bookkeeper and organizational wizardress, and

Doctors Marc Le Gras and Douglas King and Martin Lees, Dave's colleagues, who have saved thousands of children and are affable deft graceful men, and the biology scholars and professors Terry Favero and Bret Tobalske and Mike Snow, who cheerfully crammed new knowledge into me like peanut butter into an empty jar; and I commend also the American scholar J. M. Robinson, who did heroic work rescuing the Nag Hammadi codices from greedier scholars, and Doctors J. Willis Hurst and C. Richard Conti and W. Bruce Fye (what *is* it with doctors and the first-initial thing?), who together edited the invaluable text *Profiles in Cardiology* in which I swam for months like a cheerful trout, and the courteous and genial Docteur Francis Maurice Fontan of Bordeaux, France, who in 1968 figured out a way to edit the hearts of small patients with busted hearts, which I am awfully glad he did, and for which I have many gratitudes and prayers in my mouth. Thanks also to my friends the poets Kim Stafford and Pattiann Rogers and Cynthia Ozick and Barry Lopez and James Button and May Lam and Martin Flanagan and Mick Mulcrone and Joe McAvoy and David Duncan, who teach me daily by the sheen and bone of their peculiar characters, although Duncan has the most abysmal taste in fine whiskies imaginable, great a man as he is, and this reminds me that his voice is in Chapter 8, he's the man who wants to live heartish and not headish, which further reminds me to recommend, if you have not yet read it, which you must, his extraordinary book *My Story as Told by Water*, which is really astounding, one of the most substantive spiritual books I have ever read, along with everything by Primo Levi, and Annie Dillard's *For the Time Being*, and Frank McCourt's *Angela's Ashes* (I mean, really, how *can* that man have a shred of forgiveness in him after such a howling childhood?). So I assign you a little homework there if you haven't read those books; and to all the folks above, my heartfelt thanks.

Donations & Involvements

If you want to poke a little deeper than this scrawny tome can go, you might want to check out a brave woman named Leslie Morrisette, mother of the late Graham Morrisette in Chapter 9, who started an organization called the Grahamtastic Connection to put laptops with Internet connections in every pediatric bone-marrow transplant room in the United States, because her boy loved to email his buddies and web-surf and play games on our computer, and Leslie's convinced that "there are many families struggling with childhood illnesses that do not have computers and internet access and the net is a necessity to families and children battling life-threatening diseases," so if you want to help, visit www.grahamtastic.org.

Also you might, while surfing the web with money in your hand, eager to help out doctors and nurses and kids, see www. nmmc.am/eng, which is the Nork-Marash Medical Center in Yerevan, Armenia, and Nork-Marash, you will remember, is Hagop Houvaguimian's genius brainchild, which he invented from nothing and which has saved thousands of children's lives. Just visiting the site is fun; you are greeted in nine languages, which doesn't happen every day.

Providence Health Services' Heart and Vasculat Institute, bless their souls, can be webbed at www.oregon.providence. org/patients/programs/providence-heart-and-vascular-institute. The remarkable Dr. Albert Starr, now eighty-five years old and director emeritus of the institute, returned to Oregon Health Sciences University in 2011, where he is today intent on making OHSU a "center for innovation in the treatment of heart disease," as he says. See www.ohsu.edu.

Finally, with immense affection and respect, I report that Doctor Dave McIrvin and his astounding bride Linda McIrvin now run Sanctuary Camp, in Steamboat Springs,

Colorado, "a camp facility for seriously ill patients and their families from across America," says Linda. "When a person is diagnosed with a serious illness, the whole family becomes the patient. Our purpose it to provide a place for the family to be together in a therapeutic, natural environment and achieve respite from the stresses of medical care and hospitalizations." Dave and Linda also characteristically pour their energies into all sorts of projects through Sanctuary Camp: the Wounded Warriors Project, which teaches wounded veterans of America's wars to ski; Sunshine Kids, which brings children with serious diseases onto the slopes; and STARS (Steamboat Adaptive Recreational Sports), which brings people with all sorts of disabilities and damages into the crisp sky and soaring light of the mountains. See www.sanctuarycamp.us or email Linda directly at sanctuarycamp@gmail.com.

About Brian Doyle

Brian Doyle edits *Portland Magazine* at the University of Portland, in Oregon—"the best spiritual magazine in the country," according to author Annie Dillard. Doyle is the author of twelve books, among them *The Grail*, about a year in an Oregon vineyard, and the "sprawling serpentine riverine sinuous" novel *Mink River*, about an Oregon coast town; both are available from Oregon State University Press. Doyle's books have five times been finalists for the Oregon Book Award, his work has been reprinted in the annual *Best American Essays*, *Best American Science & Nature Writing*, and *Best American Spiritual Writing* anthologies, and he was awarded the 2008 Award in Literature from the American Academy of Arts and letters, "for utterly murky and inexplicable reasons," as he says.